Good Dog, Happy Baby

Also by Michael Wombacher

Integrated Dog Training:
The Commonsense Visual Guide to Training Any Dog

There's a Puppy in the House: Surviving the First Five Months

Good Dog, Happy Baby

Preparing Your Dog for the Arrival of Your Child

Michael Wombacher

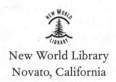

New World Library
Novato, California

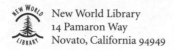
New World Library
14 Pamaron Way
Novato, California 94949

All photos are by Rose Guilbert, except where otherwise noted.
Illustrations by Bruce Henderson
Text design by Tona Pearce Myers

Library of Congress Cataloging-in-Publication

Wombacher, Michael, date.
Good dog, happy baby : preparing your dog for the arrival of your child / Michael Wombacher.
    -- Revised edition. pages cm
ISBN 978-1-60868-852-4 (paperback : alk. paper) -- ISBN 978-1-60868-853-1 (ebook)
 1. Dogs--Behavior 2. Infants. 3. Dogs--Training. I. Title.
SF433.W63 2015
636.7'0835--dc23   2015001646

First published in hardcover by New World Library in 2015
First paperback printing, February 2023
ISBN 978-1-60868-852-4
Ebook ISBN 978-1-60868-853-1
Printed in Canada on 100% postconsumer-waste recycled paper

New World Library is proud to be a Gold Certified Environmentally Responsible Publisher. Publisher certification awarded by Green Press Initiative.
www.greenpressinitiative.org

10   9   8   7   6   5   4   3   2   1

Contents

Introduction

A few weeks before I began writing this book, I sat at my desk shaking my head in exasperation. I had just hung up after a call from yet another couple who had decided to give up their dog three months after they'd had a child. "It's just too much," they told me. I had sensed the tears welling up in their eyes. "The dog pees every time we pay attention to our baby, he runs around the house and barks at her, he growls when we put her on the sofa, which he's no longer allowed on, and he seems to have generally just gone crazy." I'd explained to them everything they would have to do to correct the situation. They'd realized they simply didn't have the time. Not with two jobs and a new baby. Sadly, they gave up the dog.

Even sadder was that the entire situation would have been preventable had they started working with their dog from the day they learned they were expecting. At least twice a month, I counsel expectant parents on how to prepare their dogs for the arrival of a child, and after receiving this last phone call I decided the time had come to put advice on paper. If more people could readily access this information, I thought, perhaps fewer dogs would be given up within a few months of a baby's arrival.

With that motivation I set out to write this book. I have tried to cover every conceivable issue related to bringing a child into a home with one or more dogs. From a great deal of practical experience, I know that the actions outlined in this book work. The essential trick is taking the time to do them — sooner rather than later. Otherwise you may end up like the couple mentioned earlier and give up your dog.

Before getting to the meat of the subject, let's take a few moments to examine the cultural context of what is to follow. Perhaps the most significant thing to note is that the last fifty or so years have produced enormous changes in the social status of dogs. As late as the 1970s, it was not uncommon to find the family dog relegated to the backyard, where, it was assumed, he was happy on his own with a doghouse, a bone, and an occasional play session with his human.

Since then, dogs have transitioned from the backyard to the bedroom. In the course of that transition, dogs have taken up new niches in the shifting social landscape of their human caregivers. Among those new niches is the role of surrogate child: as women freed themselves from traditional constraints and entered the workforce, many of them postponed having children. Dogs filled the void for childless young couples, effectively becoming the first step in the building of a family. Simultaneously, dog ownership in general has increased significantly. An estimated 40 percent of American households, or 75 million, are now home to at least one dog.

Good Dog, Healthy Child

Dog ownership has skyrocketed in the last half century, and an increasing body of information illustrates the many benefits of a loving relationship with man's best friend. In fact, studies have shown that children who own dogs are less narcissistic, and they possess greater, authentic self-esteem and empathy than children who don't. Understandably such children tend to be more popular in school and are quicker to develop friendships. Dogs also offer unqualified friendship to both children and adults during stressful and lonely times.

And there's more. Dog ownership provides potential health benefits to children. For instance, in an age of increasing, chronic childhood obesity, children with dogs tend to be more active and so are less likely to undergo the ravages of this affliction. Studies have also shown that owners of dogs suffer fewer common ailments such as headaches and colds, have reduced stress levels, and experience lower heart rates and blood pressure.

All in all, when well-integrated, dogs and children make fantastic companions.

So what happens when the surrogate child is supplanted by an actual one? The seriousness of this question is highlighted by the fact that, of the approximately 4.7 million people a year who suffer dog bites in the United States, 80 percent are children under five. Doubly sobering is the fact that 80 percent of those bites are on the face. Of course, the damage is both physical and psychological, with a majority of victims experiencing some form of post–traumatic stress disorder when the bite is substantial. Additionally, most of the bites come from dogs in the victim's household and are related to seemingly harmless activities such as playing, petting, and feeding, and these dogs have no previous history of biting.[1] The obvious question for expectant parents, then, is: What can we do to protect both our child and our dog? This book is dedicated to exploring that question.

Here's how the book is organized and how it can help you. In the first chapter, you will find a questionnaire designed to help assess whether your relationship with your dog is healthy and conducive to the introduction of a new "pack member." If you find that it isn't, the Doggie Twelve-Step Program will help you get there. The chapter also discusses ways to deal with annoying canine antics and lays the groundwork for the resolution of serious behavior problems.

The first chapter is comprehensive, and I recommend that you read it in its entirety, or at least skim it, since it contains the fundamental building blocks of a wholesome relationship between you, your dog, and your new child. Of course, if your dog is perfectly well behaved already, and you feel that your relationship with him in terms of social status is well balanced and appropriate, then you might simply skim chapter 1. But I recommend that you at least peruse it just to be sure that you have dotted your i's and crossed your t's.

In the second chapter, I address a variety of behavior problems that could make introducing a child into a dog's life problematic. You can search through this chapter to locate the discussion of problems you are experiencing, or check the table of contents or the index. I'm sure you will find relevant answers here. But please bear in mind that the content of the first chapter is foundational to the behavior modification strategies outlined in the second.

In the third chapter, I share a series of pragmatic exercises designed to prepare your dog for the changes in your household that will accompany the arrival of your child. I recommend that you incorporate into your life as many of the exercises as feasible. They are designed to teach your dog to make powerful positive associations with the presence of your child. Good preparation of your dog means the day of your child's birth will represent a bump in the road, not a catastrophe.

Finally, let me say a few things about my training philosophy. On the whole, the approach I discuss in this book is a balanced one that combines the benefits of positive reinforcement with a psychological approach to dog behavior while maintaining the benefits of structure, guidance, and authority.

This approach is not "positive only" — I do not consistently discourage all forms of reprimand. This approach also operates on the presumption that a dog's psychological makeup is that of a social creature who functions best in a hierarchically structured and consistent social situation. The reason for mentioning this at the outset is that in the last twenty years a training approach known as positive-only training has become popular. Advocates of this approach insist both that dogs are not pack creatures who function best in the context of hierarchy, and that any form of reprimand other than a gentle "no," a time-out, and the removal of some desired result are tantamount to abuse. I disagree with this line of reasoning.

To be fair, this approach has been, and continues to be, a response to so-called yank-and-jerk training that dominated the training world for centuries. Harsh corrections were seen as the primary training methodologies; thankfully, in tandem with all the rights movements during the 1960s, this idea was challenged and supplanted by insights from marine mammal training, such as operant conditioning and other more humane methods. This was very much needed, but over time the pendulum has swung to an extreme degree in the opposite direction, and positive training became positive-only training.

This newer method has serious shortcomings. There is not enough room here to review them all; suffice it to say that such an approach eliminates a host of effective training strategies from the fully stocked training toolbox that all good trainers should have at their disposal. It attempts to mold the entirety of the dog and her motivations and behaviors with a training approach that represents a fraction of available approaches.

This seriously shortchanges both dog and owner. And that is doubly true in the context of this book and our attempt to ensure the seamless integration of a baby into a house with a resident dog. There is so much at stake, and limiting the range of approaches with which to address the situation, in favor of only one training philosophy, seems unfair. As a result, I have outlined a host of integrated strategies that combine positive reinforcement with psychological methods of behavior modification and appropriate compulsion, in such a way that we maximize the positive, minimize the negative, are realistic about the constraints of the situation, and focus intensely on getting results.[2]

In what follows I offer, where possible, multiple strategies, ranging from the strictly positive to the more compulsive. That way you have a range of options at your disposal and can choose the one that most closely matches

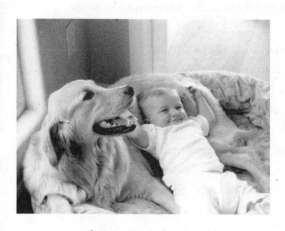

your disposition and that of your dog. Along these lines, whenever possible it is important to do everything you can to "catch your dog doing something right." In a balanced approach to dog training, we do not shy away from compulsive methods when necessary, but we are always looking for ways to reinforce positive behaviors that are the opposite of the negative behaviors we are attempting to eliminate. For instance, if your dog has a

strong habit of jumping up on you, then whenever you see him restrain himself and refrain from jumping up, be sure to immediately positively reinforce that behavior, either with lavish physical praise or a favorite treat. Again, catch him doing something right, and then bring a lot of attention to that moment in order to highlight it in your dog's mind.

On a related note, throughout the book I suggest various forms of harmless but effective ways of correcting a dog using, alternatively, a squirt bottle with water that you've set to shoot a jet stream, some Binaca breath spray (those minty little breath sprays meant to freshen the breath after lunch or coffee), taste-deterrent sprays such as Bitter Apple or Bitter Yuck (commonly used to prevent dogs from chewing furniture), or Pet Correctors (small canisters of compressed air that blasts out fairly intensely, accompanied by a loud, compressed air sound). When I suggest using a squirt bottle filled with water, please know that in the event that the water does not prove effective you may also try any of these suggestions as an alternative.

Finally, a few notes on writing style. First, there are occasions throughout this book where I repeat myself. The reason for this is twofold. Some things bear repeating simply for emphasis, and you may want to skip around this book scanning for answers to specific problems. I want to be sure that the repeated points are likely to be read by all. Additionally, there is the issue of gender. Since we have no gender-neutral pronouns available in the English language, throughout what follows I refer to both dogs and owners sometimes as "he" and sometimes as "she." That way, everyone gets equal time and no one feels left out.

So, let's dive in and see how we can prepare your dog for the arrival of a child.

Chapter One

Early Considerations

Congratulations! You're pregnant and your "pack" will soon be growing. If you're like most people, you're caught between anticipation and trepidation. You're thrilled about the arrival of your new child, and you're concerned about doing everything right. If you own a dog, certainly some of your concern revolves around him. You're probably asking yourself, "How will my dog handle this? Will he be jealous? Will he be careful?" And most important: "Is there any chance that he might bite my child?" If you're not concerned, you should be. As I have already mentioned, approximately 80 percent of dog bites happen to children under five. The purpose of this book is to help you find your way through these concerns, answer important questions, and set the stage for a warm and mutually beneficial relationship between your dog and your new child. In addition, this book addresses the difficult question of whether having the dog you have right now will be appropriate when your new child arrives.

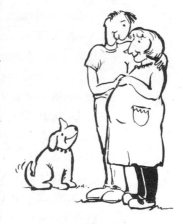

Heads Up!

Before discussing ways to ensure a smooth transition into siblinghood for your dog, it would be wise to assess whether there are any obvious potential problems looming on the horizon. Below I have provided a laundry list of questions you should ask yourself even if you're not pregnant but are simply considering the possibility. Take some time to observe your dog and answer these questions honestly. Doing so will allow you to notice any red flags and give you a head start in resolving problems if they do indeed exist. If you find no behavior problems, well, you're in good shape, aren't you? In that case feel free to merely skim the Doggie Twelve-Step Program in this chapter; skip chapter 2, "Addressing and Resolving Potential Behavior Problems"; and go straight to the final chapter, "A Seamless Transition," which outlines how best to ease your dog through the transition to life with a child.

Okay, here goes.

- Does your dog like children?
- Has he been exposed to them on a consistent basis? If not, why not? If it's simply for lack of opportunity, then now would be a good time to start exposing him to children while you closely observe his responses. Is he shy and intimidated? Is he suspicious? Is he overexuberant and pushy?
- What is your dog's general disposition? Is he sensitive to or fearful of novel stimulation such as loud noises, sudden movements, and rough handling? Is he hand shy? Is he emotionally dependent on you and generally spoiled? Is he afraid of being left alone? Is he pushy and demanding?
- Does your dog exhibit problematic behaviors? Some examples: Does he bark at you for attention? Does he jump up on you and your guests as a form of greeting? Does he steal food from tables or beg

incessantly at dinnertime? And how does your dog relate generally to food and toys or other objects he considers his own? Does he need his own area in which to eat or chew on his favorite toys? Can you take anything away from him at any time without the slightest form of resistance? If your dog does offer resistance, what kind is it? Does he simply tense up and look at you out of the corner of his eye? Does he growl? Does he actually snap and bite? If your dog has furniture rights, do you have trouble removing him from the furniture? Do you have trouble getting him to move out of your way if he's resting somewhere? Is your dog overterritorial? Does he threaten your guests? Does he bark excessively? Does your dog understand obedience commands? If so, how well does he obey them?

If you have more than one dog in your household, ask yourself the preceding questions about each dog and then consider the following ones as well:

- How do your dogs get along together?
- Do they ever fight? If so, over what? Over food? Over toys? Over special places? Over you? Have they injured each other?
- Do they compete for your attention?
- Is it clear who is the dominant dog in your pack? Do you hold the leadership position in your pack?

This last issue is of utmost importance. Dogs are pack animals and, by their very nature, *crave* structure and authority or, in short, leadership. (By the way, this is true of children also.) If a dog does not perceive leadership in his environment, he will assume that the role, by default, is his. As political scientists will tell you: power, like nature, abhors a vacuum. A dog who perceives himself as leader in his human environment can be the source of significant problems, including many of those implied by the earlier questions.

If you're planning to bring a child into a household in which your dog is confused about his status or thinks he is the leader, whatever problems you are having now are highly likely to increase significantly. Because introducing a baby will change the structure of your dog's pack, he may feel the need to assert himself over any new members and reevaluate his relationship with existing members. Clearly, you don't want your dog asserting himself over your new baby. Even if your dog is not the assertive type and tends more in the fearful direction, the perception of a lack of effective leadership may exacerbate such fear and can contribute to a behavioral disposition simply known as fear-aggression. Effective leadership, then, results in not only the resolution of any behavior problems but also the seamless introduction of a new child to your pack.

WHAT IS LEADERSHIP?

Being your dog's leader does not mean being a bully. True leadership has to do with confidence, the ability to give direction, and the willingness to follow through on directions given. It also has to do with being trustworthy and reasonable in the demands one makes. A great general does not lead because he can beat up his soldiers. He leads because he embodies certain qualities that make others want to follow his lead. Your embodiment of leadership qualities will make your dog look to you for direction more than any act of brute force ever could. And should you be concerned that your dog will no longer like you if you take charge of his life, rest assured that the person who puts the most pressure on a dog, *in a fair way*, gets the lion's share of that dog's love, affection, and respect.

With that in mind, I'm going to set forth by outlining my Doggie Twelve-Step Program. This is a rank-management program designed to establish you in the leadership position, and it forms a springboard for discussing the resolution of any potential problems. If you don't feel you're experiencing any problems with your dog, the application of this program may reveal areas of difficulty you were not aware of. Moreover, a great many elements of this routine should be implemented even if you're having no trouble with your dog, simply because they ensure good and safe behavior in all situations, especially those including children. Also, as you read through this program, you may find that some of the things discussed apply directly to your situation and others don't. Feel free to implement what makes sense in your context, and don't worry about what doesn't. If you find that your dog is perfectly well mannered in relation to all the things outlined in the program, consider yourself lucky and, by all means, move along through the rest of this book.

The Doggie Twelve-Step Program

This program ensures that your dog is receiving a coherent message about her social status in your household. It combines a variety of psychological and physical methodologies that appeal to her canine sensibilities and will help her become and remain a well-behaved and smoothly integrated member of your growing household.

1. Learn to Earn

In a pack situation the leader dog largely gets whatever he wants, anytime he wants it, from anyone he wants. This is in keeping with his position and makes perfect sense in that context. If in the human context the same thing happens — that is, the dog gets whatever he wants and no demands are placed on him — he simply has no choice but to conclude that he must be in charge. After all, if he weren't the leader why would everyone be so compliant? It follows that since he views himself as being in charge, he also views himself

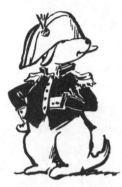

as having a variety of rights — rights that could lead him to act in inappropriate ways. The first step in adjusting the dog's view of himself, then, is to demote him from royalty to commoner and insist that he earn his living.

What this means in real time is that for every nice thing you do for your dog, he must do something for you first. For example, before you give him so much as a pat on the head you should ask him to comply with an obedience command, even if it's something as simple as "sit." If he doesn't do it, you gently but quickly make him. Any other nice things you do for him, such as feeding him, taking him

A legend in his own mind.

for a walk, or playing with him, should be preceded by some type of demand. It could be anything — even a cute trick. Just be sure that it's not always the same demand. In other words, don't always ask him for the same old sit. Be sure to ask him for downs (that is, to lie down), for stands, for a short bit of heeling, or even, as I said, a silly trick. It doesn't really matter what it is so long as he does something for you before you do something for him.

The point? To get your dog to exercise impulse control and to look to you for direction. "Pattern training," or always asking for the same thing, defeats the purpose of what you're trying to do. If the dog is pattern trained he's merely running the pattern and not truly looking to you for direction, which is precisely the habit you want to get him into. *He should get used to exercising impulse control and looking to you for direction in all things that are important to him.* This will begin to position you as leader in your dog's mind. For most dogs this little routine goes a long way in ensuring a proper attitude toward their owners. Some dogs aren't quite that easy, however, and require a little extra effort.

WHY RUN THE SHOW?

Dogs who are used to taking direction from their owners in relation to things that are important to them are easy to guide into new behaviors. Propriety and respect are second nature to such dogs, and this means a bigger, more inclusive life for everyone.

If you're experiencing more serious attitude problems with your dog (if she's the pushy and demanding type), it's also useful to spend some time during the day actively ignoring her. Nothing gets a dog's attention like simply ignoring her. During a period of time when your dog is used to having your attention, simply cold-shoulder her. This means *do not look at, speak to, or touch her.* If she comes over to pester you for attention, either get up and walk off, run her through a bunch of obedience drills, or simply tell her to go away. Put a little theater into it and act annoyed to drive the point home. If your dog is the superpushy type and refuses to depart despite your theatrics, a squirt from a water bottle (if water doesn't bother her, try a taste deterrent such as Bitter Apple spray, or a breath spray like Binaca) right on her nose and mouth should convince her to depart.

For those pushy dogs used to demanding their owners' undivided attention most of the time, this kind of treatment may come as a shock. In fact, they may even go through a short period of depression, moping around with a "hangdog" look. If this happens to your dog, don't worry. Not only is this perfectly normal, but it is actually a good sign, as well. It simply means your dog knows that "the times, they are a changin'," and the upset likely will pass within three to seven days. Typically the more indulged the dog was, the longer the period of depression, but every dog invariably gets over it as she adjusts to the new regime and comes to terms with the new situation. From this much more solid foundation a whole new relationship can be built.

I have found that this part of the program — turning one's attention into a valued resource rather than having it taken for granted when dealing with a dog with attitude — is often the most emotionally challenging part for owners. In fact, in most cases it is more difficult for the owner than the dog. But trust me: once you are on the other side of this, your dog will love and respect you dramatically more, not less, than she did before, and I promise that you will not break her spirit. On the contrary, you'll have transformed the very foundation of your relationship into one of trust and respect and will be well positioned to teach her how to live with you and your new child in a positive and integrated way, which will make your partnership more fulfilling for both of you.

PLAY HARD TO GET

Playing hard to get is extremely effective in getting a dog's attention. Few things will snap his head around like temporarily depriving him of your affection. Make yourself into a valued resource, and your dog will see you in an entirely new light.

Believe me, simply pulling off this part of the rank-management program will cause your dog to look at you in an entirely new way. He will immediately begin to respect you and, yes, love you more. Always bear in mind that dogs crave structure and leadership, and that *the person who puts the most pressure on a dog, in a fair way, gets the lion's share of the dog's love, affection, and respect.*

2. Teach and Practice Obedience Exercises

A great deal of what I outline here presumes that your dog understands obedience commands. If he doesn't, you should begin teaching them immediately. Every dog's vocabulary, in my view, should include at a minimum the commands sit, down, stay, come, and off. Additionally, your dog should walk nicely on the leash and be generally attentive to you. More advanced commands include directing the dog to stand-stay (to hold a stay in a standing still position), heel, and perform emergency stops at a distance. I assure you that most every dog can learn these commands regardless of age, breed, or previous history. The only exception would be a geriatric dog who is essentially senile and physically incapacitated.

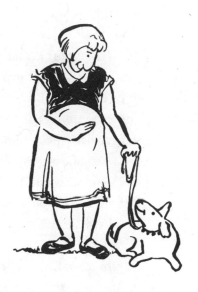

A HAILING FREQUENCY

"Open a channel!" These were Captain Jean-Luc Picard's famous words when contacting an alien species. Obedience training opens a channel of communication between you and your dog, one that facilitates interspecies relationships and understanding. "Make it so!"

While this isn't the place for an extensive discussion of teaching obedience commands, I'll share one self-control exercise that I view as indispensable and which is surprisingly easy to teach. It's the sixty-minute down-stay.
Now, you might be thinking, "Sixty minutes — no way! Not possible!" But
it's easier than you may think. Select a one-hour period during the evening
— perhaps while watching your favorite television program — put your
dog on a leash and place him in a down-stay near you. Put one foot on the
leash so he can't get far if he decides to move, have the handle in your hand,
and then relax and watch your program. Your dog may lie down and sleep
if he likes, or he can watch TV if he's that sort, but he is not to get up *under
any circumstances*. If he tries to get up, which he inevitably will in the beginning, quickly place him back in his down-stay and start over. Most dogs get
it rather quickly; but *no matter how long it takes, stay with it*. Once he does
it in one situation, try it in another one. And then another. Imagine how
helpful this will be when you're trying to get something done with your new
child, like sitting down and nursing your baby with your dog lying calmly at
your side.

In general, obedience exercises are crucial to the development of a proper
relationship with any dog, but they are utterly indispensable if you're planning to have your dog live with a new child in the household. If your dog
has no understanding of obedience commands, he will most likely end up
spending a great deal of time isolated from the new social situation, and, as
I said, this is something you want to avoid at all costs. Isolation will only
teach your dog that his life took a radical turn for the worse the day your
baby arrived. This means that if your dog's understanding of obedience commands is limited, now might be a good time to hire a trainer or attend some
classes.

3. Control Feeding Arrangements

Food is the primary survival resource. Because of this I have often said that food is to dogs what money is to people. Whoever controls the food potentially commands a great deal of respect and authority. As a general rule, the higher-ranking individuals among wolf and dog packs have access to the premium pieces of food, while others have to wait their turn in accordance with

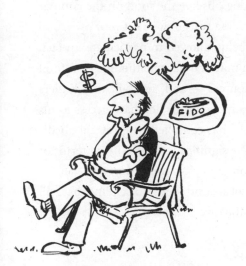

Food is to dogs what money is to people.

their social status; the lowest-ranking pack members usually have to settle for scraps and leftovers. This orientation is deeply ingrained in your dog, and you can avail yourself of it when asserting your leadership in a nonconfrontational way.

The following routine will allow you to send a strong message to your dog about control of the food and, by extension, about your authority. Begin by preparing your dog's meal in front of him in as enticing a way as possible. Go ahead, be theatrical. The goal is to get him as worked up as you can over his impending meal. However, just when he thinks he's about to be fed, take his dish and place it on a counter were he cannot get it. Then walk over to your own dining area, put your dog in a down-stay or tether him to a piece of furniture nearby and proceed to eat something yourself. If your now somewhat frustrated dog begins to pester you by barking or whining, a quick "quiet" command, enforced if necessary with a quick squirt from a water bottle, should settle him down. Convey to him in no uncertain terms that he is not to bother you while you are eating. Then take your time and enjoy your food. Build as much tension in the dog in relation to the food as possible. Only when you are completely finished with your meal should you return to the kitchen, take his food off the counter, show it to him, and ask him to comply with a couple of obedience commands. Only then should you finally feed him.

The point of all this is to let your dog observe the food on the counter were he cannot get it. Then he should observe you going to eat your own food and take note of the fact that he's not being allowed to participate. In fact, he has to keep a respectful distance and now can have neither his own food nor yours because you control both resources — and, after all, pack leaders eat first. Not until you are good and ready may your dog have access to his food, and even that happens only after he has complied with several obedience commands and earned his meal. The significance of all this in terms of social status will definitely not be lost on your dog. Moreover, this exercise will teach your dog significant self-control around food, a discipline that will be a great asset once you have a child in the mix.

4. Control Sleeping and Resting Areas

One of the ways a higher-ranking dog may choose to assert himself is by controlling space with his body. In his own mind his status affords him the right to sleep or rest anywhere he likes and to demand that others move away from his favorite spots. He may also insist that if he is lying in a certain spot, no one may come within a few feet of his "critical zone," the area around him that a dog tends to view as an extension of himself. One clear sign that your dog has issues with social status is if he growls, snaps, or even shows milder forms of resistance toward you when you approach or try to move him from his favorite places. In fact, this is one of the most common situations in which owners get bitten by their dogs. If your dog has bitten or threatened to bite you in this context, please read the section "Dealing with a Dangerous Dog," on page 92. The best way to respond to this, and an important aspect of sending the right message regarding rank to your dog, is to control access to all furniture, beds, and favorite resting places. The benefits of having such control when a youngster is around should be evident.

There are different ways you can approach this, and which one you choose is completely up to you. You can eliminate all furniture rights for your dog. Or you can teach him that he's allowed on the furniture only with your invitation, and that he must get off the moment you demand it. Or you can even teach him that he's allowed only on certain pieces of furniture, and only at your invitation. If you choose one of the latter options, I recommend eliminating furniture rights altogether in the short term and using this as a default position. You can then reintroduce furniture rights with your invitation once this is solidly understood.

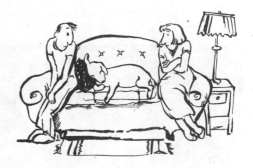

Access to sleeping and resting areas may be controlled in a number of ways. You can reprimand your dog with a sharp "no" or "off" (use your squirt bottle or simply physically shoo the dog off in order to enforce this, if necessary) every time he begins to get up on a piece of furniture. Or you can close the doors to those areas where he likes to make himself at home, booby-trap furniture items with sheets of tinfoil or with ScatMats (rubber mats emitting mild static electricity), or simply keep the dog leashed to you in order to deny him access to these places. This last strategy is often effective simply because it denies the dog any freedom of movement other than where you direct him, which firmly puts you in a leadership position. Letting him drag a leash around the house — an extension of the idea of keeping him leashed to you — is another effective way to control his movements. It allows you to simply use the end of the leash to pull him off the sofa or bed rather than having to grab for him.

If your dog has favorite places to sleep, and you sense that he's attached to them to a fault (in other words, he might defend them), it's a good idea to deny him access to these places as well. *This might seem harsh, but you don't want your dog having any sense of ownership over special places.* An easy way to deny him access to those places is to ask him to sleep in a different location each night. Tethering or restricting him to a different spot every evening is a good way to accomplish this. Now don't get me wrong. The idea is not to make him uncomfortable, only to make him lose his sense of possession of favorite places. By all means, make sure he's cozy. Just control where that takes place.

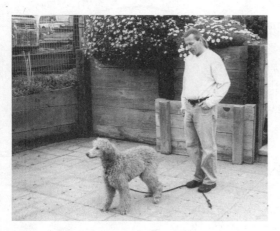

Letting your dog drag a leash around is a great way to get a handle on him.

Once your dog has relinquished furniture rights for some period of time and has resigned himself to this, you may, as stated earlier, reintroduce them on your terms *if you so desire*. There are a number of ways to do this. You can teach him to come up on an "invitation only" basis. The invitation can be a simple phrase such as "c'mon up," accompanied by a pat on the sofa. You can also do what I do. I have a special blanket that I spread out on the sofa when I want my dog up with me. This keeps him from getting any dirt on the furniture, and it's also a visual cue for permission to come up. When he sees the blanket come out, he knows he's about to be invited up. I still say, "C'mon up," and pat the blanket just to be sure that he doesn't confuse that blanket with others (this is especially important with a baby around). By controlling your dog's behavior in this way, you can control access to your furniture while being able to snuggle with your dog on the sofa as well. In short, allow your dog access to the furniture on a "sublet" basis only, and you can have your cake and eat it too.

A RENTAL AGREEMENT

Possession is nine-tenths of the law, as the old saying goes. Make sure you possess the rights to all furniture and resting places; and if you do allow your dog access to these areas, make sure it's on a "sublet" basis only.

5. Make the Dog Move Out of Your Way

Another way to control space and assert your role as leader is to simply make your dog move out of your way as you are walking around your home. As

mentioned, many pushy dogs like to control space with their bodies. This means you may often find yours lying right in the middle of major thorough-fares in your house such as hallways, doorways, and any other areas that see a lot of traffic. Often, not wanting to bother the dog, you may find your-self simply walking around her, thinking that you should just let her have her space. This can be a mis-take. It potentially sends her the signal that you are

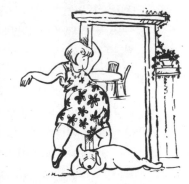

deferring to her authority by avoiding contact with her and respecting her
"critical zone" when she's resting. What you should do instead is simply ask
her to get up and move.

Of course, if your dog is sleeping you should have the courtesy to wake
her up first. The command I use to ask the dog to move out of my way is simply: "Excuse me." Approach your dog, clap your hands, and then, in a happy
tone, say, "Excuse me." If the dog does not move out of your way relatively
quickly, you can gently nudge her with your foot to demand that she move.
You should look for multiple opportunities each day to ask her to move out
of your way. Eventually, if you have practiced this exercise consistently, when
your dog sees you coming she will simply get up and move without being
asked. If your dog has bitten or threatened to bite you in this context, please
read the section "Dealing with a Dangerous Dog," on page 92.

6. Control Access to Narrow Openings

When you pass through a door or other
narrow passageway, you should go first
and your dog should wait to be asked to
follow. This is not only an important exercise from a safety standpoint (you don't
want your dog dragging you out the door
when you've got a newborn in your arms),
but it has certain psychological implications as well. Part of the pack leader's job
is to lead the pack into new and productive
situations. If your dog bolts through the
doorway every time he sees a crack of light,
he is playing that role and taking charge.

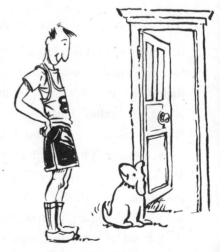

Wait, please!

In this context it's important to understand that, for your dog, the doorway represents a huge change of consciousness. To put it differently, from your perspective the two of you are merely going for a walk, but from your dog's perspective the two of you are going hunting. In short, your dog is moving from the "den" to the "hunt" — two modes that are about as far apart in his psychic and sensory experience as possible. The entirety of your dog's awareness goes from a state of being almost totally dormant to a state of extreme alertness and stimulation in a matter of a few moments. No wonder he's bouncing around at the front door. Keep in mind that, for your dog, there are few things as pleasurable as hunting, an activity rooted in the prey instinct and about as primal as it gets. For this reason, he should understand 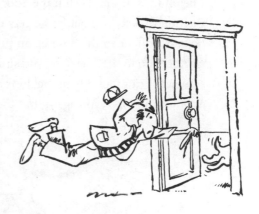 that he needs to go through you to access that state of consciousness. To put it differently: you should become the doorway through which he must pass in order to have access to any of the things that are important to him, including the hunt.

TAKE CHARGE

Taking control of every aspect of your dog's life will cause him to have tremendous confidence in you. Not only that, but it will also allow you to safely integrate your dog into every aspect of your life, making the relationship more fulfilling for both of you.

There are several effective and easy ways to teach your dog not to pass through the doorway before you. The first is to simply open the door just a hair as your dog is approaching it and, as he makes a dash for it, shut it in his face abruptly (not *on* his face, please!). Timing is of the essence here. Obviously, you should avoid trapping the dog's head in the door and hurting him. The point is to simply shut the door in front of him, loudly if possible, just a fraction of a second before he gets there, in order to startle him. As soon as he backs off, open the door again just a hair. Most likely your dog will make another run for it. If he does, you simply repeat the procedure. Now he will be somewhat cautious. Open the door again, this time a bit farther. If he makes another run for it, you again shut the door in front of him.

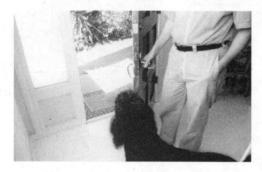

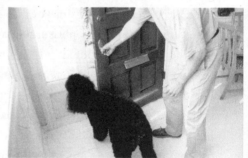

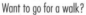

Want to go for a walk?   Not so fast.

By this time the dog will likely be a little bit confused. You continue to open the door ever farther and tempt your dog to run out, repeating this procedure until he simply does not rush the door. Likely there will be a moment where the dog, in utter confusion, will look at you as if to say, "Hey, what's going on here?" This is your moment of opportunity. While he's looking at you in confusion, ask him to sit. Very likely you will find that he responds promptly. Confusion is a great state in which to learn. Your dog does not know what's going on, and he's looking to you for an answer. You, being the leader, provide the answer, which is simply: "Sit." Once your dog understands that he should sit at the doorway, be sure not to let him out until he hears a verbal invitation, such as "Okay, let's go" from you. Soon he'll learn that a doorway is a dangerous place if you haven't passed through it first, and he'll wait for your direction before proceeding.

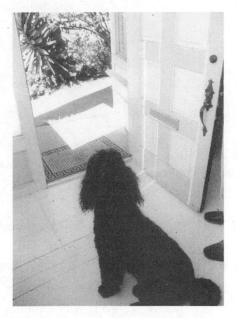

That's better.

Another, more direct way to teach him the same concept is to simply attach his leash to his training collar. I prefer pinch collars, which, despite their ferocious appearance, are actually among the most humane training devices available. When properly fitted and used, they reduce the level of force you use on your dog by about 95 percent and almost entirely eliminate any possibility of injuring him (see appendix). Open the door in the way described earlier, and if he makes a run for it, pull back promptly at the moment his nose passes the threshold of the doorway. I feel justified snapping the leash, if necessary, in this situation, since it represents such a significant safety concern for you, your child, and your dog. If he rushes at the door again, repeat the procedure. Again, once he inhibits himself, ask him to "sit," and when he's settled tell him, "Let's go."

Either one of these two procedures will teach your dog to look to you before passing through the doorway, but I prefer the first since it involves no real discomfort to the dog. With some dogs, the really headstrong type, using both techniques in succession is necessary to really make the effects foolproof.

WHAT IS A CORRECTION?

One form of correction is a nudge with a leash attached to a training collar. By a nudge I don't mean pulling and restraining a dog or swinging him around like a tetherball. A nudge is a quick snap and release on the leash (kind of like snapping a towel when you were a kid) primarily designed to get the dog's attention. A proper training collar will ensure that a little nudge will go a long way. (See the appendix for information regarding training equipment.) The level of force you use should be determined by the sensitivity of your dog, but the best policy is to find the level of correction that gets the message across after one to two repetitions.

Finally, if you want your dog to consistently pay close attention to you, always ask him for compliance with a different command before permitting him to go out the door. In other words, instead of always asking him to sit, occasionally ask him to lie down, or to stand, or anything else you can think of. Never knowing what's coming next keeps him looking to you for direction, which, of course, is the point.

7. Do Not Let the Dog Pull Ahead of You on the Leash

Unless you're training for the Iditarod, your dog should learn not to pull on her leash when out for a walk. Not only should she learn to accompany you without exerting any tension on the leash, but she should also remain largely oriented toward you. In far too many cases the owner is — from the point of view of the dog — little more than a piece of dead weight on the end of the leash to be dragged around. Trying to walk a dog like this can be not only annoying but also dangerous, especially if you also have a newborn in a stroller or baby carrier. Moreover, what the dog is gleaning from the situation should be obvious: she, not you, is leading the parade. Definitely the wrong impression! Your dog should learn to walk on a loose lead while keeping at least half of one eyeball on you at all times. This does not mean she has to walk alongside you in a formal heel position, but it does mean she should to pay attention to you. This reorientation of the dog is achieved through something I call the "pay-attention game."

Begin by putting a training collar (see the appendix for a discussion of pinch collars) or a chest-leading harness (a harness with the leash clip on the chest) on your dog. If you are using a pinch collar it is important that it be nice and snug. Loose pinch collars have a nasty tendency to fall off, since part of what holds them together is a little tension between the links. More-over, the looser the collar, the firmer the 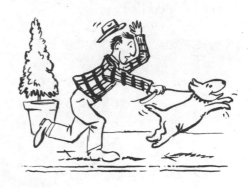 correction you must deliver in order for the collar to function as designed. Finally, if a pinch collar is too loose, the prongs, instead of pinching slightly the way they're supposed to, can actually jab the dog's neck, a decidedly undesirable outcome. Since the whole point of the pinch collar is to take as much physical force as possible out of training, a loose collar would be counterproductive.

Once the collar is fit snugly, you attach your six-foot leash to it. Then insert your thumb through the leash handle and take up a little slack, creating a loop in your hand. If your dog is not familiar with the pinch collar, the first thing you must do is introduce it gently in order to let her know

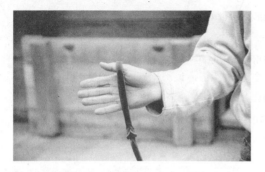

Put your thumb through the leash handle.

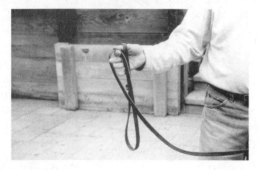

Take up some slack.

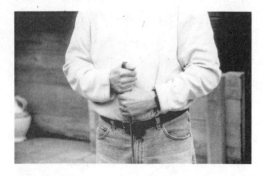

Drop and stop.

there is something new happening on her neck today. Start your introductory exercise by simply walking with the dog. As you see that she is beginning to forge ahead and is either pulling on the leash or simply failing to pay at least some attention to you, suddenly drop the slack in the lead, grab the leash handle with both hands like a baseball bat, hold it firmly to your belly button, and stop. Since your dog is not paying attention, she will continue to walk and will suddenly hit the end of the leash with the force of her own momentum. This will deliver a minor correction and will likely cause her to turn around and look at you with a startled expression.

At this point, encourage her to come back to you with a pat on your thigh and, once she's near you, praise her and resume your walk, being sure to take up the slack in the leash as you did before. Then, simply repeat the procedure. You will find that soon your dog will stay a little closer to you and pay a little more attention to what you're up to. Ultimately when you stop, your dog will automatically stop as well. This little exercise gently gets the dog used to the pinch collar and teaches her the fundamental concepts of the pay-attention game, which are: don't pull, and keep an eye on me. Once this happens, you're ready for the next step.

Begin by walking with your dog as you did a moment ago. When you see that the dog is forging ahead, it's time to take action. However, now when you drop the slack in the leash, instead of simply stopping you turn around and, *without warning your dog*, march briskly in the opposite direction. Again, the dog will hit the end of the leash; and this time not only will she hit it with the force of her own momentum, but she will also feel your momentum going in the opposite direction. If you completed the previous exercise, your dog most likely will have caught on to this trick and will know what to do to avoid a more noticeable correction. But if not, the correction she receives in this exercise will give her a strong incentive to keep a close eye on you and follow you wherever you're going.

Of course, once your dog is near you, you should praise her wildly. This will teach her that being near you and paying attention is the "safe" thing to do, and being out there and not paying attention permits potentially unpleasant things to happen. Pretty soon you'll find that it's nearly impossible to lose your dog. When you've arrived at this point, start exposing your dog to increasingly distracting situations in order to test her willingness to pull on the leash.

To ensure the correct performance of this exercise, I'll emphasize three extremely important points: (a) drop the slack in the leash just *before* you turn, (b) don't issue any verbal warning to your dog (this would indicate to her that you will always alert her to changes in direction, and that she has no responsibility to stay alert to changes herself), and (c) make sure you do not yank her after she's made her turn. Once your dog learns to avoid the correction, she'll walk near you without exerting any tension on the leash and will also shadow your movements most of the time. In other words, you've now

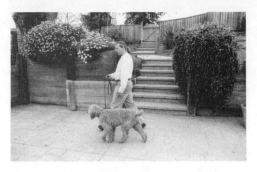

1. Begin by walking with your dog.

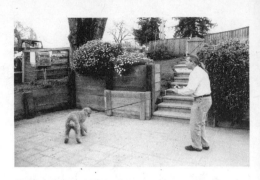

2. When she forges ahead or fails to pay attention, just stop. Do not yank!

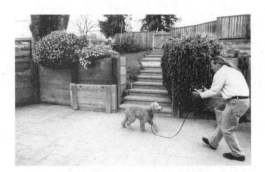

3. Immediately encourage your dog to return to you. Praise her when she does.

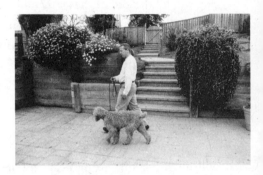

4. Once again, begin walking with your dog.

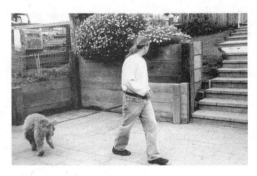

5. This time when your dog forges ahead, drop the slack in the leash, as shown above, lock it into your belly button, and briskly march in the opposite direction. Do not yank!

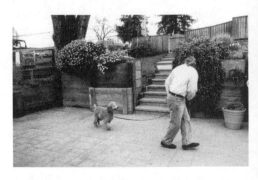

6. And, of course, enthusiastically praise your dog as she catches up with you.

become relevant and she's following you, not dragging you down the street. In this context, it doesn't matter whether the dog is walking slightly ahead of you, slightly behind you, or a little out to the side. *What matters is that she's paying attention to you.* When your dog walks ahead of you, but stays right with you even when you turn in the opposite direction, who's the leader? Clearly you are! Moreover, your walk with her is now not only much safer and more pleasurable but also a powerful context in which you assert your leadership role.

8. Do Not Let the Dog Jump Up on You as a Form of Greeting

Jumping up, while usually a friendly gesture of greeting, is not only pushy and dominant but also presents obvious problems when you are trying to navigate your day with a small child in tow. Your dog should learn that the fastest way for her to get your attention and affection when greeting you is to keep all four feet on the ground. This can be accomplished by simply using a variety of different approaches.

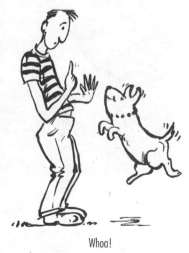

Whoa!

First, you can try simply turning your back on your dog when she jumps up on you, depriving her of the very thing she wants — your attention. When, faced with your back, she gets down, turn around and begin to give her attention. If she jumps up again, repeat. For dogs who learn from this method, it usually takes between three and five turns before they get the idea — four feet on the ground brings the dog the attention she wants, two feet off the ground removes it. If it takes many more than five repetitions, then this approach probably won't work for you, and pursuing it much longer will simply result in scratch marks on your back. If that is the case, you should try the other methods outlined here.

The next one involves taking a squirt bottle that will allow you to shoot a jet of water, fill it, and *hide it behind your back* so the dog cannot see it. Then, enter the area where your dog would be likely to jump up on you and, when she jumps, give her a quick squirt right on the nose and mouth while loudly saying "off". (more on this command in a moment). Then, just as quickly, return the bottle to its hiding place behind your back. This will likely come as a great shock to her. As she's recovering from her shock, actually encourage her to jump up on you again by speaking to her in a sweet voice, patting your chest, and doing anything that will tempt her to repeat this maneuver. In human terms, this is called "entrapment," and it might seem inherently

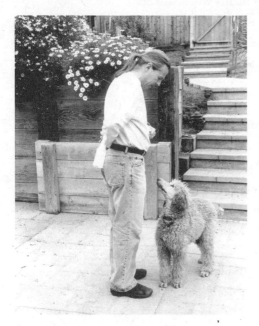

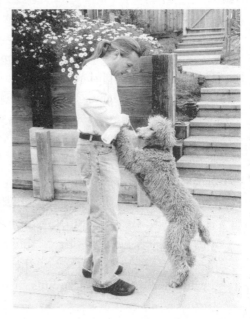

Be sure to conceal the squirt bottle behind your back.   Not so fast.

unfair. However, in training terms it is called a "set up" and is wonderfully useful. In this case, the point is to set her up and then teach her that there is simply no reason for her to jump regardless of what you're doing. Children habitually do all sorts of things that tempt dogs to jump on them, and your dog should learn to restrain herself so that she doesn't inadvertently injure your child.

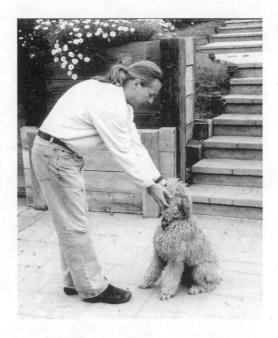

Practice this exercise diligently in relation to both your guests and yourself (squirt her with water or give her a blast from your canister of compressed air — the Pet Corrector — when she jumps on them or you), and soon you'll notice that your dog is beginning to

That's better.

control herself. *Do not overlook this positive development!* Too many dogs get attention only when they're acting out in annoying ways, while good behavior hardly gets a second look. Once you see that your dog is restraining herself, you should find a way to *reinforce this opposite behavior* — that is, when she is not jumping up. In fact, the second she makes the decision not to jump on you, or perhaps even to sit, bend down and reward her with attention, praise, and perhaps even a handy and well-timed treat. In this way she learns that all the praise, attention, and affection that she is looking for will come to her automatically if she simply keeps four feet on the ground. It also teaches her to maintain a certain degree of social distance, even in highly charged situations.

A CANINE HANDSHAKE

Your dog jumping up on people is the canine equivalent of you going up
to a perfect stranger, wildly throwing your arms around him, and giving
him a kiss as a form of greeting. While friendly and well intentioned, that
greeting would be totally inappropriate and would most likely get you
beaten up or arrested. A handshake is what's called for, and the canine
equivalent of a handshake is a sit-stay.

If your dog happens to jump up on you when you don't have a squirt
bottle handy, you can use one of a number of other maneuvers to surprise
her. For example, when she jumps up, grab both of her feet, one firmly in
each hand, and hold them away from your body as if you were dancing with
her. While you're doing this, apply some firm pressure to her paws and simultaneously walk her backward. This will likely make her uncomfortable, and she'll struggle to get away from you. Continue to hold her for a few moments while she's struggling, and then finally release her. She'll soon catch on.

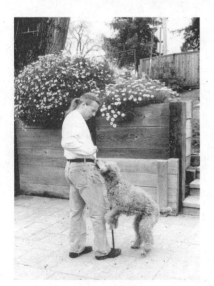

Standing on the leash is simple and efficient.

Another method involves simply grabbing your dog's muzzle as she jumps up on you, squeezing it shut, and then gently but firmly pushing her into a sitting position on the ground. Of course, the moment she's sitting begin petting and praising her.

Alternatively, if she's on a leash, you can lower it so that some of it is on the ground, and then stand on that section. This way, every time your dog begins to jump up she'll get about three inches off the ground and hit the end of the leash — a built-in, perfectly timed correction. This will almost always automatically guide her back to a sitting position, where you can tell her what a good girl she is.

Whichever approach you use, be consistent and diligent, and soon you'll find that your jumping problem has dissipated and will ultimately disappear altogether.

9. Do Not Let the Dog Take Food without Your Permission

As we saw earlier, food is the primary survival resource, and control of the food resource is symbolic and highly meaningful to your dog. Too many dogs are far too pushy around food, sometimes being so bold as to grab things right out of people's hands. Clearly this is inappropriate and even dangerous if a small child is involved. (If your dog has bitten or threatened to bite you in relation to food and objects, please read the section "Dealing with a Dangerous Dog," on page 92.)

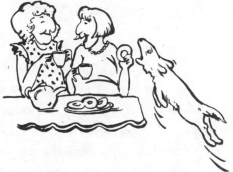

One of the most important things to teach your dog, then, is a solid "off" command. To do this you need a handful of yummy treats and a squirt bottle filled with either water or Bitter Apple spray (what you use depends on your dog's sensitivity). Begin by holding a treat in front of him and saying, "Take it." Your dog should promptly come over and take the treat, at which point you'll offer him another, saying, "Take it" again. Once more he'll come over and grab the treat. Repeat this procedure five or six times, until your dog is really anticipating a treat. Then suddenly, without warning, as he approaches the next treat, give him the command "off" instead of "take it." If the dog continues to go for the treat — and most likely he will, since he does not know the "off" command — quickly spray him on the nose with whatever is in your squirt bottle, preferably water in the beginning.

KEEP YOUR PAWS TO YOURSELF, PLEASE

If you allow your dog to take food from you without your permission, it will be easy for him to conclude that he can do the same with your child. This, in turn, will teach him that your child is an easy mark for a food mugging, and he will most likely conclude that Junior is a lower-ranking pack member. For this reason, your dog may conclude that he has the right to reprimand your child; and dog reprimands usually take the form of a quick bite. Stop trouble before it starts. No pushy behavior around food, please.

Your dog will likely back off with a shocked expression on his face (if he doesn't, that is the time to consider escalating from water to a taste deterrent such as Bitter Apple spray or a similar product). As soon as he does this you praise him enthusiastically and offer him the treat again with the command "take it." It may take a few repetitions for him to become totally confident about taking the treat once more; but when he does, you repeat the procedure. Give him five or six treats in a row prefaced by the "take it" invitation, and then suddenly give him the command "off" and follow up with the spray *if needed*. You'll be amazed at how fast your dog will learn that it's okay to take the treat when given the "take it" command, and that when he hears the "off" command he should immediately back off. Most likely, after three to five iterations your dog will hear the command "off" and quickly back off without needing to be sprayed.

There are a couple of important points to mention here. First, *timing is of the essence.* You must pause for a moment between issuing the "off" command and spraying your dog. This moment is his window of opportunity. He needs a moment to process the command and comply. This allows him a chance to avoid the correction with the squirt bottle, and that, of course, is the point. The word *off* is his cue that if he backs out of the situation immediately, nothing unpleasant will happen to him.

Second, it is important to be sneaky with the bottle — don't make it too obvious. Hiding it behind your back and bringing it out just as you're about to spray him is the best tactic. Then, as fast as it came out, the bottle should disappear again so that your dog has only a second or so of exposure to it. You want him to understand that the essential thing is the command "off," not the fact that you have a bottle. If your dog learns that the bottle is the deterrent he will forever be looking for it and, if he doesn't see it, may be tempted to continue with the behavior. This is called "equipment orientation," and you don't want him weighing his choices, basing his decision on whether he sees a bottle in your hand. Instead, you want him to think you potentially have that squirt bottle on you at all times. Once he believes this, he will stop testing you.

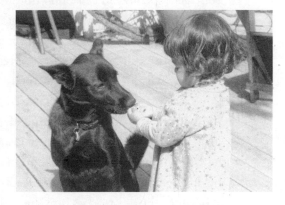

Photo: Jane Reed

The next step involves continuing with this exercise until you cannot get the dog to take the treat after the command "off" has been issued. When he has a solid understanding of this, then go to the next step by throwing a treat on the floor. Again, initially let him have three or four treats prefaced with the command "take it," and then issue the "off" command once more. If he does not immediately retreat, he gets sprayed. Keep your timing in mind. Give him a moment to respond before you spray him. Once your dog has a solid understanding of these exercises, then use the "off" command in various contexts around the house. For example, you can be standing in the kitchen working on dinner and suddenly throw a piece of food on the floor. When your dog goes to get it, you issue the command "off," and if he leaves it alone he's a good boy; if he doesn't he gets sprayed.

Once your dog has internalized this and is no longer taking food without your permission, you can ramp up the "off" command to another level. Put him on his leash and bring along whatever training equipment you are using; then take him outside with a handful of treats. While you are walking, suddenly and without warning throw a treat on the ground a few feet in front of him where he can see it. Once again, for the first three to five times simply let him have it. Then suddenly give the command "off" as he begins to approach the next treat. If he does not immediately turn away, give him a quick snap of the leash — just enough to get his attention. Most likely at this moment he will, with a surprised expression, turn his head toward you. The moment he does, give him a treat. *You do this even if you had to give him a correction.*

Over time this teaches him that, when he hears "off," he should not only get off whatever he was focused on, but that he should look at you as well. You are now giving him two powerful motivations to take his eyes off whatever they're focused on. First, is the risk of a correction that he has learned he can avoid by backing away from whatever he's interested in. Second, is his reward for giving you his attention once he hears the "off" command. That's about as black and white as you can make it.

Once he's learned the concept of "off" in a training context, it's time to start using it in a variety of situations. Until your dog has thoroughly internalized this command, be prepared either with your squirt bottle (hidden behind your back) or with a leash and training collar, so that, should he test you, you can correct him. However, if you're consistent with this for even a short period, you'll soon find that you won't need squirt bottles, training collars, or any other gimmicks. Your dog will simply have learned the command, and you will have it available to you in a great variety of situations.

In this context, also teach your dog that food on surfaces such as coffee tables and kitchen counters is off limits as well. Set tempting morsels out where he can see them, and pretend not to watch. Of course, when he makes a move on the items you should give him a loud "off" and a squirt with your squirt bottle.

Which brings me to the "atomic off." This is the PhD program of the "off" command. Take a plate of food, your food, something really wonderful that your dog simply won't be able to

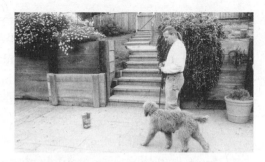

The "off" command. For the purpose of these pictures, I used a bag rather than throwing a treat.

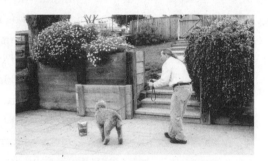

As your dog approaches, give the command "off," and if she doesn't comply, give a short snap.

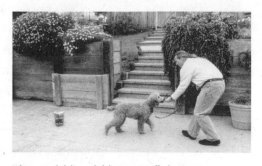

When your slightly startled dog returns, offer her a treat.

resist, and place it in the middle of your living room floor. Then take him by the collar in a calm and matter-of-fact way, walk him over to it, pointing it out and telling him, in a commanding but not harsh tone, "off." Then walk him away to some other part of the room and let him go. Now, the idea is that since you've been working hard on the "off" command in the way described earlier, and he's heard you say "off" in relation to the plate of food, he shouldn't think of going near it.

In reality, this is probably not going to happen just yet. A plate of food on the floor is simply too tempting. What's more likely is that shortly after you release your dog, he'll find his way back to the food and make a run at it. Of course you or an accomplice will be lying in wait, preferably in an area where

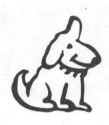

you won't be obvious to the dog. In one hand you should have a squirt bottle, and in the other a shake can (an empty soda can with five or six pennies in it and a piece of tape across the top to keep them from falling out) or a Pet Corrector (a canister of compressed air). When your dog arrives near the food and his intent is clear, you loudly surprise and severely startle him. Rattle your shake can, squirt him on the nose, blast the Pet Corrector, and strongly reprimand him. If you've done this properly he should hightail it out of the area. The idea is to stun him and convince him that going after something once you've told him "off" is a poor strategy.

To assess whether your reprimand was effective, you should leave the plate of food out for the rest of the night. If your dog makes another run at it he's telling you that you weren't sufficiently convincing the first time around; you need to ramp up the level of your reprimand. If you've done this properly your dog will not only avoid that plate of food for the rest of the night, but he'll also learn to take your "off" commands much more seriously in the future — a lesson that will be extremely helpful once there is a baby in your life.

The fact is that every household with young children I've ever visited is inherently chaotic. There are toys, food, and a variety of other items randomly strewn all over the place. Having a solid "off" command available to you will be extraordinarily useful in managing your dog and preventing him from getting into things that he shouldn't be into or which could be dangerous for him. In fact, without an effective "off" command you'll find yourself either endlessly and futilely screaming "no" at your dog or simply locking him up. And in this context it would become easy for your dog to associate being locked up or yelled at with the presence of your child, a scenario you want to avoid at all costs.

In short, teaching a powerful "off" command opens many lines of communication with your dog and is fundamental to many of the exercises that follow in this book. Paradoxically, having a strong "off" command will also allow you to give your dog more freedom, in due course, because you will easily be able to instruct him in what he may do and what he should stay away from, a capacity that will be exceedingly helpful as you instruct your dog in how to properly relate to your child.

10. Control the Games the Dog Is Allowed to Play

As we've already seen, a dog who has unrestricted access to resources can easily develop an attitude problem. In this context both toys and games are valuable resources and should be controlled. If you're experiencing attitude problems with your dog, which might be expressed by the dog endlessly bringing you her toys and demanding a game, guarding toys, or just making it difficult for you to take them from her, begin by removing all her toys from the environment. This means that you have total control over this resource. But that's not the only consideration. Soon you'll have children's toys scattered about, and having dog toys haphazardly thrown in the mix can lead to a host of problems (which I'll address in a subsequent section).

At any rate, now that your dog no longer has indiscriminate access to her toys, and to the games that she can play with them, you are in a position to control this resource and initiate games with her *if you so choose*. She has to go through you in order to have access to this source of fun. As a side note: avoid chase games altogether. Such games teach your dog that she is faster and stronger than you or your child, and this is information she can definitely live without.

FUN AND GAMES

Fun and games are serious business to your dog. Be her portal to pleasure by making her go through you to get them.

Let's see what it means, in practical terms, when *you initiate, control, and end games* at your discretion. If you like playing fetch with your dog, bring out a toy when you're ready to play, *not when she demands it*, and show it to her. Before you throw it, ask her to comply with an obedience command. It can be anything, but make sure you don't throw the toy unless your dog has performed the command — nicely. When she brings the toy back and gives it to you (if she doesn't give it up, use the "off" command), ask her for a different command and demand compliance before you throw it again.

Continue to do this throughout your play session; and when you've had enough, end the game by using a cue phrase such as "that's enough" and simply putting the toy away. If your dog continues to pester you for more, you might respond by running her through short obedience drills. A mind-numbing routine of sit-down-sit-down-stay-sit-stay-down and so on should do the trick. She'll soon get the idea and leave you alone. In sum, then, whatever games you play with your dog, be sure they all follow this pattern: you initiate, control, and end them.

In relation to this, if your dog is the pushy and demanding type, then roughhousing, wrestling, and other physically competitive games should be temporarily eliminated. As you progress in this program, and you sense that your dog has adopted a more respectful attitude toward you, these games may be reintroduced so long as the rules outlined earlier are followed. For example, if you're roughhousing with your dog, you should, first, give her a verbal cue that a game is about to begin, such as "Okay, let's play." Without this cue, roughhousing should not be allowed, since you don't want your dog eventually initiating roughhousing sessions with your child. Second, take a break every thirty to forty-five seconds, demand a number of obedience commands, and then resume the game.

During the course of your roughhousing, you should also repeatedly put the dog in a submissive position — that is, on her side or back, with you hovering over her. At this time you should handle her in slightly annoying ways to teach her to accept childlike and even inappropriate handling. The idea, of course, is to teach her to take such handling in stride. In relation to this, I will talk later about teaching your child to appropriately handle your dog.

The point of these exercises is simply to build tolerance in your dog so that she can be prepared for the kind of handling your child may inadvertently dish out. In this context, any rebellious behavior on your dog's part should immediately be met with a prompt cessation of the fun, a firm verbal reprimand, and a string of obedience commands. Also, during the course of all this, you should *be sure that your dog never uses her teeth* on you in any way. Whether gentle or hard, any contact of your dog's teeth with human skin should be strongly discouraged.

If your dog does make such contact, immediately either say "ouch" in a high-pitched tone as if you'd been hurt and quickly pull your hand or arm away or, if this does not work after a few repetitions, grab her muzzle and squeeze it shut (but not so hard as to catch her tongue or lips between her teeth and hurt her), issue a sharp verbal reprimand, and temporarily cease the game. Spraying her with a squirt bottle can also deter this behavior. In short, you should have *a zero-tolerance biting policy*; with a child on the way, the reasons should be obvious. If you work on this diligently, by the time your child arrives your dog should have learned never to put her mouth on human skin for any reason, period.

Moreover, you may have read that tug-of-war games with dogs should be avoided altogether because they encourage dominance and, as a result, potentially aggressive behavior. My view is that this is a half-truth. On the one hand, if you cannot control the game, then definitely don't play it. However, if you can control the game it can be helpful in asserting your authority over your dog in a context of fun and partnership.

Let's explore how you can play tug-of-war and have it support the fundamental task of the rank-management program. As I've already said, you should always be the one who initiates the game. Grab the toy and approach the dog, teasing her with it. Give her whatever verbal cue you've decided on to let her know you're now ready to play. As she begins to show interest, ask her to comply with an obedience command. The moment she does so, offer her the toy and begin playing tug-of-war. It's okay to play as hard and rough as you want, *provided your dog's teeth are not touching you in any way* — allow no reckless or careless biting, please. In fact, to make it difficult for your dog to

Photo: Belinda Levinson

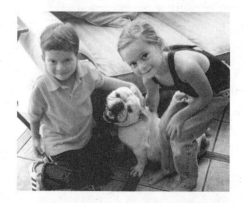

inadvertently bite you, move the toy quickly and unpredictably and immediately issue a verbal reprimand if she does bite. Then, run her through a
few obedience commands before continuing. If she repeatedly makes contact
nonetheless, then, after three infractions, end the game.

The point is to teach the dog to be *very careful* even when she's totally
worked up, and that there are consequences (game over — sorry!) for failing
to exercise restraint. On the other hand, as long as your dog is not recklessly
biting, continue to play with her as hard as you want, suddenly commanding
"off" at thirty- to forty-five-second intervals. This should not be a problem if
you've developed some proficiency in the exercises I've described here.

If your dog does not immediately release the toy, spray her in the mouth
with water, Binaca breath spray, or Bitter Apple spray or give her a quick blast
from the Pet Corrector. One of these will almost always make her give up the toy
instantly. Once she gives it up, promptly issue a command like "sit" or "down."
The moment she executes this command, once again offer her the toy and resume playing. Continue like this for as long as you like, being sure to demand
an obedience command every thirty to forty-five seconds. Played in this way the
tug-of-war game actually supports your rank-management program by teaching your dog that you control the entire event. She learns that recklessness is
unacceptable, and that by virtue of your authority, an "off" command is all you
need in order to gain possession of the precious tug toy. The beauty of this game
is that it not only reinforces your leadership status but also teaches your dog to
take direction from you when she's extremely excited. And it helps channel her
intense play and prey drives into compliance with obedience commands.

11. Do Not Let the Dog Take Positions above You

In many ways, dogs, complex and multidimensional though they are, are also
relatively simple, straightforward creatures. This is particularly true in relation

to physical postures. A dog will tend to perceive individuals who are physically above him as potentially above him in social status as well (this is not always true, but it's true often enough to warrant our attention). Conversely, he will tend to regard anyone physically beneath him as socially beneath him. You can use this simple calculus to your advantage when addressing issues of social status with your dog by doing what you can to prevent your dog from taking up positions above you.

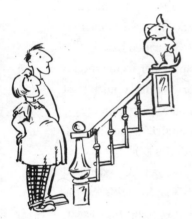

A dog can assume a position above you in a variety of ways. He can jump on top of you when you're lying down. He can climb into your lap and make himself at home there without an invitation. He can run up a staircase ahead of you and stand at the top looking down at you as you follow him. If you have an interior staircase in your house, he might also find the stair or landing that is elevated just above everyone's head and make that a favorite resting place — a vantage point from which he can survey his domain.

A PROPER PERSPECTIVE

Make your dog answer to a "higher power" by taking up positions above him. Looking down on him in this manner means he will have to look up at you, and such a posture will do his outlook on your relationship a world of good.

Taking up positions above you is a meaningful activity for your dog that should be curbed when you need to shift his perception of his place in your pack. Doing so is a nonconfrontational means to assert your authority in a way that is intelligible to your dog's canine sensibilities. For instance, if you're walking up a set of stairs, ask your dog to hold a sit-stay at the bottom of the staircase, and call him once you're at the top. If you're descending the stairs, don't let him bolt down, but instead have him walk down alongside you. And if your dog is seeking positions in your house such as landings on interior staircases that allow him a vantage point above your head and shoulders, he should be denied access to these areas.

If he likes to climb on top of you and lie in your lap uninvited, this is a variation on the same theme. While endearing, it is a pushy and demanding behavior that should be eliminated or at the very least put under your control. So, each time your dog attempts to climb up on you, issue a firm "off" command and shove him off, backing it up with a squirt bottle if necessary. As with furniture rights (see pages 12–15), once your dog no longer takes it upon himself to hop into your lap, you may invite him there if you so desire. The key here is that the choice is yours, not his.

While these responses to your dog taking up positions above or on top of you might seem a little excessive, please keep in mind that in their absence it may be easy for him to inappropriately assume superior positions in relation to your child and, consequently, conclude that he can treat your child as a lower-ranking pack member.

In this context it's important to remember, as I mentioned earlier, that initially when you increase the social distance between you and your dog by doing exercises like this, he might sulk and act depressed for a time. While this can be difficult to take, I assure you that he'll get over it within three to seven days and then come to terms with his new status in your life. And the fact is, by the time your baby arrives, it will be extremely important for your dog to understand his appropriate place in your pack. Bear in mind that if you attempt to implement social changes abruptly after your baby arrives, it's likely that your dog will associate these changes with that arrival and come to take a dim view of the newcomer.

12. Groom and Handle Your Dog Regularly

It almost goes without saying that you should be able to handle your dog in any way you see fit. Yet some dogs become quite sensitive to having certain areas of their bodies handled and may even become aggressive if you insist on touching them there (if your dog has bitten or threatened to bite you in this context, please read the section "Dealing with a Dangerous Dog," on page 92). It makes sense to be sure that your dog is completely relaxed about being touched in a number of different ways.

There are many areas on a dog's body to pay special attention to. First, a dog has what are known as *socially sensitive* areas. Primary among these are the upper back and shoulder areas, as well as the back of the neck. Others include the underside of his chin and neck, and his hindquarters. Additionally, many dogs extremely dislike having their paws handled. Ask any vet or groomer, and they will readily attest to the number of bites generated by touching a dog's feet.

In order to significantly develop your dog's level of tolerance for being touched in these areas, groom and handle him regularly as an indispensable part of preparing him for the arrival of your baby. Doing so will not only condition him to accept this type of handling, but it will also help you assert your physical authority over him in a potentially pleasurable way. If he is sensitive to such handling, you must go through routines of systematic desensitization in order to teach him to take it all in stride. These routines are discussed in detail a little farther on.

TRUST AND RESPECT

Trust and respect are the cornerstones of any healthy relationship. Handling your dog regularly will teach him to trust that nothing unpleasant will befall him and to respect your right to subject him to such handling.

In addition to touching your dog across the entirety of his body, you should be able to place him in various vulnerable positions gently yet firmly and have him accept such handling in stride. If your dog is small to medium size he should allow you to cradle him like a baby in your arms — upside-down with your hand on his belly. If he struggles against you, firmly demand that he stay there by clamping down on him and issuing a moderately intense reprimand such as "uh-uh-uh." Once he relaxes, you may gently stroke him, teaching him that the end of resistance brings pleasure and the reduction of stress. You may even offer him a small, yummy treat if he's having a particularly difficult time with it all. Similarly, your dog should allow you to place him on his side on the floor and crouch over him, with your hands gently pinning him to the floor, until you decide to release him. And again, if he relaxes, gently stroke him and perhaps even reward him with a little treat.

Additionally, once you have him in this position, you should be able to give him a thorough and pleasurable body exam and massage. Any mouthing or biting should be met with a firm reprimand as described earlier. These actions, from the perspective of your dog, are significant in relation to social status. As we saw earlier, if you are able to assert yourself by being physically above your dog while placing him in submissive and vulnerable positions, he will understand that your position is socially superior to his. So not only are you teaching your dog to accept various forms of handling without stress, but you have also found one more way to contribute to the coherent message about social status and pack dynamics that you send to your dog. (Note: For more on this subject, please see the videos on my website at www.doggone good.org/training-video-series/).

An important detail in this context is that you should never attempt these handling exercises with a dog who believes that he is firmly entrenched in a leadership position. Doing so could lead to a bite! Before attempting any such exercises with a dog like this, be sure that you have diligently implemented every other aspect of this program for some time and have seen a significant change in his demeanor. If you are still concerned that your dog might bite or threaten to bite you in this context, please read the section "Dealing with a Dangerous Dog," on page 92.

As I mentioned before, this rank-management program is designed to build a foundation on which you can resolve most potential behavior problems in your dog long before the arrival of your child. And even if you're not experiencing any real problems with your dog, the rules set forth here are almost indispensable if you're going to have a small child around. After all, do you want your dog jumping up on everyone, stealing food, refusing to obey commands, climbing all over the furniture, and demanding games from you or your child? Of course not. A dog like this will inevitably be relegated to the fringe of your life rather than being integrated as part of the family unit.

If you are experiencing behavior problems such as the ones listed at the beginning of this chapter, or any others, you may find that simply implementing the program outlined here diminishes or even entirely eliminates them. This is because, once your dog understands his appropriate social position, he will no longer feel compelled to act out as if it were his role to run your household. If confusion about social status is driving his problem behaviors, these behaviors may dissolve of their own accord once the issue of status has been dealt with. If they don't, at least you've laid the foundation for dissolving them. In the next chapter, we'll look at a number of exercises that will help eliminate a variety of problem behaviors that would make having your dog in the presence of a child a bad idea.

Summary of the Doggie Twelve-Step Program

1. Play hard to get, and make your dog work for a living.
2. Teach and practice obedience exercises. Include long down-stays in his daily routine.
3. Control feeding arrangements so that you eat before your dog *and he knows it!*
4. Control sleeping and resting areas.
5. Make the dog move out of your way at least ten to fifteen times a day.
6. Control access to narrow openings. Make your dog look to you for direction when embarking on any new ventures.
7. Do not let your dog pull ahead of you on the leash. Be a leader and lead!
8. Do not let your dog jump all over you or anyone else as a form of greeting.
9. Do not let your dog take food from you or any place in the home without your permission. Teach a solid "off" command.
10. Control the games your dog is allowed to play. Remember, you initiate, control, and end all games.
11. Do not let your dog take positions above you.
12. Groom and handle your dog regularly.

A Final Thought

Please understand that dogs crave structure, guidance, and authority. So, the person who puts the most pressure and demands on a dog *in a fair way* will get the lion's share of the dog's love, affection, and respect. That should be you! This chapter has shown you how to put yourself in that position if you aren't already there. By being your dog's leader you are well positioned to guide him into his new life with your child.

Chapter Two

Addressing and Resolving Potential Behavior Problems

If you reread the list of questions raised at the beginning of the previous chapter, you'll find that many problematic issues are addressed directly by implementing the rank-management program. For example, if your dog was pushy and demanding, if he was jumping up on you, begging incessantly at the table, climbing all over the furniture, or pulling you down the street as if he were a sled dog, all this should have changed once you started applying the principles of rank management, since the principles directly address these issues. If these unacceptable behaviors haven't been resolved, then we must conclude that you haven't yet implemented the program properly, and so you might want to revisit that chapter.

In this chapter we'll take a look at what's left over. Specifically, I'll address the following questions: What if my dog doesn't like children? What if my dog is afraid of sudden movements, loud noises, or any disruption of his immediate environment? What if my dog is snappy and reactive (that is, he acts out in ways that are undesirable) to being touched in certain ways? What if he's afraid of being left alone and is generally emotionally dependent? What if he's possessive of toys or food? What if my dog barks excessively? What if he's overprotective? What if I have several dogs and they don't get along together?

Let's investigate these questions and come up with some solutions. Please keep in mind, though, that in order for the solutions outlined in this chapter to truly work, it's necessary to first implement the rank-management program described in chapter 1. That is the foundation. Without that foundation in place, taking the next steps will be like trying to build a house in quicksand, and it's likely that what is discussed here will produce, at best, marginal results. After all, you can't build a building without a foundation, and rank management is the foundation of a comprehensive and thorough approach to behavior modification.

Additionally, please be aware that the solutions provided here for issues that potentially involve aggression are primarily designed for dogs with aggression problems that could be described as mild to moderate. If you would describe your dog's problem as somewhere between moderate and severe, please read the section "Dealing with a Dangerous Dog," on page 92. Bearing all this in mind, let's get started.

What If My Dog Doesn't Like Children?

There are many reasons dogs don't like children, but most of them revolve around a lack of early socialization with them. Additionally, children's noisiness and generally unpredictable nature make many dogs apprehensive, and some unpleasant experience with a child in a dog's history may contribute to his general aversion. (If your dog has bitten or threatened to bite children, please read the section "Dealing with a Dangerous Dog," on page 92.) Whatever the case, the solution is the same: you must gradually get the dog used to the presence of children in increments he can tolerate. The goal, of course, is to teach him, first, that children are not a threat but a potential source of pleasurable experiences, and second, that there are acceptable ways of interacting with them.

There are two types of canine temperament to consider here: the fearful one and the dominant, pushy, and overexuberant one. Let's start with the more common type, the fearful one. Whenever you deal with issues of fear in a dog, you must prove to him systematically that "the only thing to fear is fear itself." Since your dog doesn't speak English, you can't simply say to him, "Hey, don't sweat it, no one is going to hurt you here." Instead you must prove to him through repeated experience that there's nothing to worry about. What this means practically is that you must expose him to levels of the offending stimulus (that is, children) that he can tolerate and help him connect that experience to something positive. This approach is known as "systematic desensitization" and is key to dealing with all sorts of fear-based behavior issues. Be aware that approaches using

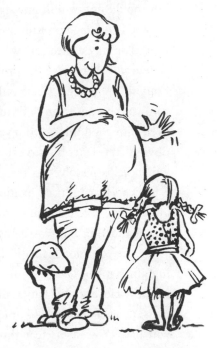

systematic desensitization may take a significant amount of time. Don't be impatient here. Slow, incremental progress is what you're looking for, not overnight results. Sometimes systematic desensitization can take months to produce solid results, and trying to rush it will only set you back. All the more reason to get started sooner rather than later.

Now, let's take a look at how you can make something like this work. The first thing you'll need to do is find some kids. This is often easier said than done, since not many moms will let you use their child as a training distraction for your dog. What I usually suggest to my clients is that they find an area where children are commonly present, such as a school or playground.

Once you find such an area, position yourself with your dog at some distance from the kids. At this distance, the dog should be aware of the children but should not exhibit any signs of fear. Once there, simply ask your dog to sit, and begin feeding him treats. (If your dog is not normally excited about food, skipping a meal or two and bringing out killer treats like hot dogs or cheese will likely solve the problem.) It's important that, during this training exercise, the dog get treats only while he's aware of the children in the environment, because you're trying to get him to associate the presence of children with good things from you. This serves several purposes. First and most obvious, it teaches him to expect something good in the presence of children, which helps dissolve his fear; and second, it puts his attention on you and relaxes his fear-induced fixation on the kids. In other words, it takes his focus away from something he's worried about and puts it on something he views as a comforting and reassuring presence, you.

Once your dog is relatively at ease with this arrangement and not showing any signs of fear, it's time to move a little closer to the children. Be sure to move closer only in increments your dog can tolerate. You want to *avoid crossing his fear threshold at all costs*, because this will only set you back. If you have crossed his fear threshold, move farther out, to a previous position that he was able to handle. When you've found the right position, repeat the procedure. Once you've got your dog's attention focused on you and the treats, begin asking him to comply with obedience commands. The more he's focused on you and has something to do, the less he'll worry about the kids. If at any point you see that your dog is beginning to become anxious about the children, go ahead and put some distance between you and them. Again, you want to be sure not to cross your dog's fear threshold and make him feel trapped by forcing too much on him too fast.

Keep repeating this procedure, always in amounts that your dog can tolerate, and eventually you'll find yourselves near the children. How long this will take depends on two things: the level of fear in your dog and the frequency of your outings with him. The more you go out with him, the faster he will get over it (nonetheless, it could take weeks to months, so please be patient). As you find yourselves getting closer and closer to the children, inevitably a child will want to come up and say hello to your dog. What you do at this time will be a judgment call. As already stated, if your dog has a propensity to bite in situations in which he's not entirely comfortable, read the section "Dealing with a Dangerous Dog," on page 92, before proceeding with this chapter.

Another factor to consider — concerning the child who wants to interact with your dog — is the child. Is he or she old enough to follow your directions when relating to your dog? If not, then you might just say that your dog is scared of children and pass on the interaction. On the other hand, if your dog is not inclined to bite and has been making good progress with these exercises, you might give the child several treats and ask him or her to offer them to your dog. *Tell the child not to attempt to pet your dog but to allow the dog to reach for the treat.* If you see that your dog is experiencing significant resistance to the whole idea, then abort the exercise. If not, then allow him to take treats from the child. If you're nervous about this aspect of the exercise, try finding a fenced-in playground where you can locate yourself on one side of the fence with your dog and have kids give your dog treats from the other side. This way, everyone is safe, and progress can be made a lot faster and with significantly less tension.

Once your dog has reached the stage where he will accept treats from one or more children through the fence — if you have found that he needs this — in a relaxed manner, you're making great progress in dealing with his fear. But take your time before you have children give him treats without the benefit of the fence. When your dog is readily taking treats from children and you've gotten to the point where the fence is no longer necessary, you want to be sure to give proper instructions to the children concerning how best to interact with and touch your dog. First, ask them not to approach the dog but to allow the dog to approach them. Additionally, instruct them not to bend over your dog, hug him, or pet him on top of his head. Have them stand with their side to the dog, reach out their hand, and, *if your dog is okay with it*, pet him under his chin and on the underside of his neck. This will appear much less domineering and threatening to your dog and will do a lot to put him at ease. Also, ask them to move slowly and deliberately rather than with sudden and sharp movements. If you get this far you're in pretty good shape. But don't rest here. Keep doing these exercises until your dog shows absolutely no fear of children.

   If you've been working near the same school or playground until now, try going to a new situation and see if what your dog has learned transfers to that situation. If not, you may have to backtrack a little in the new situation, until the dog gets comfortable in that one. When that's done, find another and so on. I cannot overemphasize the importance of frequency in relation to these exercises. You simply cannot do them too often. In fact, you should continue to do them even after you have your child, since at some point your little one is going to be bringing home little friends. "Too much is never enough" should be your guiding philosophy here, so keep working.

LITTLE BY LITTLE

I often tell my clients that in dog training, progress is always made in increments. What this means is that progress is usually not made in great leaps and bounds but in tiny steps. Nowhere is this truer than in approaches using systematic desensitization. Ironically, working slowly will produce results faster than trying to rush the lessons, which will almost always set you back.

If your dog's issue isn't fear, but is instead his pushy and dominant or overexuberant behavior, you should follow a different approach. First, consider whether your dog is getting sufficient exercise. Lack of exercise is a leading contributor to problem behaviors. There is a great deal of truth to the adage "Tired dogs are good dogs." In a well-exercised dog there is simply less energy left to throw around. In addition, obedience training is indispensable, and you should have implemented the rank-management program outlined in chapter 1. If your dog doesn't view you as leader, and doesn't understand obedience commands, you'll have practically no chance of teaching him to approach children appropriately — that is, without relating to them in a dominant or pushy fashion. On the other hand, once these elements are in place you should have an easy time of it.

In the same way described earlier, begin by bringing your dog into situations where children are present. Starting at a distance at which the children don't provide too much of a distraction, begin working your dog by using his obedience commands (which he should already know). The most important commands to focus on are sit, down, and stay. Be sure your dog is aware of the children, but that they don't provide too much of a distraction. Also, be sure your approach to training is fun and positive for your dog. You don't want him to associate the presence of children with harsh obedience exercises. Once your dog performs his commands reliably — on the first command and without corrections — at whatever distance you started with, try working him a little closer to the children. When he's okay with that, move closer still. Eventually you should be able to work your dog while close to children.

If the children begin showing an interest in your dog, hand them a few treats and have them ask him to comply with his obedience commands. If your dog suddenly won't obey, demand the behavior from him yourself. And of course, if he starts jumping or lunging you should give him a collar correction or spritz on the nose with water before placing him immediately back in a sit-stay or a down-stay. Doing this consistently will teach your dog to associate the presence of children with a particular type of behavior: obedient. This is called *situational learning*. In other words, your dog will begin to associate a particular situation (that is, being around children) with obedience exercises, sometimes demanded by you and sometimes by the kids. If he also learns that performing obedience commands for kids will often produce treats, he will soon develop a positive outlook on the entire situation. In short, when your dog sees kids, he's going to think that sit, down, and stay will mean treats and affection, and so he will soon start offering these behaviors on his own. What could be better than that?

In both of these situations you are teaching your dog a new set of expectations and responses in the presence of children. Once these expectations are internalized, the likelihood of having trouble with him around kids will be radically diminished. Once again, the more you practice in the beginning, the better. And while you'll need to do less of this as your dog gets accustomed to it, it's always good to make this a part of his daily or weekly routine. This is your best insurance policy against any future problems.

What If My Dog Is Afraid of, or Aggressive in Response to, Any Disruption of His Immediate Environment?

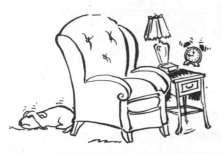

The answer to this question is essentially the same as to the previous one: your dog is in need of some systematic desensitization. In other words, he must get used to stimuli such as sudden movements and loud noises in slow, steady increments that he can handle. Again, the dog's responses can be divided into essentially two types: fearful, and pushy or dominant. If your dog has bitten or threatened to bite in this context, please read the section "Dealing with a Dangerous Dog," on page 92.

With a shy dog, the approach is identical to what I've just outlined: Bring the dog into the presence of the offending stimulus, whether it is a certain type of noise or movement or any other disruption, in doses he can handle without generating a fearful response. Then begin desensitizing him by giving him treats in conjunction with the appearance of that stimulus. In other words, teach him to associate the presence of the stimulus with something wonderful from you, and add small increments of the stimulus as the dog's ability to handle it increases. Here, too, take your time and always allow the dog room to back out of a situation if he feels threatened. Having him focused on you via obedience commands will decrease the likelihood of a fearful response, simply because a good part of his attention will be on you and not on the fear-provoking stimulus.

ATTENTION EQUALS ENERGY

If your dog's attention is focused on something he's worried about, all his energy is available to flow in that direction and will feed his fear. If you can shift some of his attention to you via obedience commands and positive rewards, it will drain a good bit of his energy away from the fear and shift it to something comforting and familiar — you, your requests, and yummy rewards. Additionally, it will put the entire experience in a positive framework.

If your dog's response to novel stimulation is to lunge, bark, or react in a pushy and assertive way, here, too, you should expose him to the stimulation in increments that do not make him reactive, and you should try to associate it with treats. However, you will most likely also have to sharply reprimand him for outbursts. In fact, I feel that if the dog has not been effectively corrected for his outbursts he may never learn that you really don't like them, even if you're teaching him to build a new set of associations. It's important to, at least a few times, put the dog in a situation that will guarantee an outburst and then to effectively correct him for it. I have already mentioned that one of the best ways to reprimand a dog without physical force is a squirt bottle filled with water. Alternatively, the Pet Corrector or Binaca breath spray or other taste deterrents will also work well with most dogs.

By communicating your disapproval of the behavior to your dog, you will help him understand where the behavior boundary is, as well as cause him to inhibit his response, putting an initial break in it. Once that's done and his inhibition increases in response to the behavior boundary, you are in a much better position to teach him a new set of responses. As an example, let's say your dog is reactive — he jumps or barks — when a guest suddenly gets up from the sofa. The moment he makes a reactive move, you should squirt him on the nose and mouth with Bitter Apple spray or give him a snap on the collar and strongly tell him "off."

Set this situation up as often as feasible and continue to reprimand your dog until he begins to inhibit himself. However, simple inhibition is not enough. In my view the problem isn't truly resolved until you can successfully undermine the core motivation that caused your dog to act out in the first place, by teaching him a new set of associations through positive reinforcement — through connecting something wonderful (such as a treat) to the offending stimulus. Continuing with the same example, now that your dog's level of reactivity to your guest is on the decline as a result of your reprimands, you should begin giving the dog a treat every time the person gets up. Soon, he'll forget about why he was upset in the first place and simply be anticipating his treat.

This approach applies to any item to which your dog is reactive, such as skateboards, bicycles, grocery carts, garbage trucks, and so on. Only when he's solidly conditioned to expect something positive in relation to the offending event, and you've had no outbursts for at least six weeks, should you consider the behavior resolved. And as your dog gets increasingly conditioned to the new set of associations, you can begin phasing out the treats. He will have learned that the sudden movements or loud noises present no threat to him, and that outbursts won't be tolerated. Here, too, you want to practice these routines as often as possible and continue to do so even when there is no longer an apparent problem. "Too much is never enough" is a good motto here.

What If My Dog Is Sensitive and Reactive to Being Touched in Certain Ways?

Again, systematic desensitization is the solution. You want to teach your dog to associate the handling with something positive and, through the course of repeated experiences, to learn to trust that kind of touching. If your dog has bitten or threatened to bite you in this context, please read the section "Dealing with a Dangerous Dog," on page 92. If your dog has not gone this far but you think he may at some point, please read on.

With a dog who is sensitive to having certain body parts touched, you should initiate an interaction by simply giving him a few treats. The best treats are those that he can continue to nibble and chew on while you're pursuing the exercise. Hot dogs or string cheese are excellent choices. Simply hold the entire treat in your hand and continue to feed it out to him as he nibbles away at it. Once he's focused on the treat and busy consuming it, *slowly* move your other hand toward whatever area is sensitive.

If at any point you sense that your dog is becoming wary, back off and simply hold your hand on or near an area where he is aware of it but not in any way reactive or even suspicious. Also, briefly remove the treats, teaching him that tolerating the touch on or near the sensitive area is directly related to receiving a treat. Restart the exercise by returning his attention to the treat and beginning to move your hand toward the sensitive area again. In most cases it will not take too many iterations before your dog ignores that hand and continues to take treats. As he does this, move your hand ever so slowly and gently closer to his sensitive area, until you are actually touching it. Once you've touched him and held the touch for a few moments, remove both your hand and the treats from your dog.

At this point, he will likely stare at the hand that had the treats in it, eagerly awaiting more. After letting his anticipation build for a few moments, again present the hand with the treat in it. While he's focused on it, slowly bring your other hand to the sensitive area again. Continue touching him there for a few moments and then remove both hands. Repeat this procedure until your dog becomes comfortable with the whole routine. Most dogs will learn relatively quickly to ignore the hand that's touching them. At this point, start adding speed to the exercise: begin moving your treat-free hand in more quickly, really reaching for your dog's sensitive area, as he continues to focus on the treat and his trust in the exercise builds. Continue increasing your speed until you can move your hand toward your dog's sensitive area at the same speed someone might use when suddenly reaching out to pet him. Throughout this time continue to present the treat to the dog at least a few seconds *before* your hand actually touches him, so that more of his focus is on the treat than on being touched.

Once this routine is solidly established, start changing the pattern by shortening the increment of time between getting the dog focused on the treat and touching him. If the dog was focused on the treat for ten seconds before you touched him, you should now cut that back to nine. Then cut it back to eight and seven and so on until there is only a one-second interval between the time the dog starts getting his treat and the time you reach for him (that is, quickly). Ultimately the day will come when you can present the treat to your dog at the moment you reach for him. Because he will at this point have had dozens to hundreds of exposures to this exercise, he will be thoroughly relaxed about it and will have learned to ignore the hand reaching for him. Spend some time repeating this step over and over until the dog is perfectly habituated to it.

The next step involves *reaching for him first* and then presenting the treat. At first, the time increment between reaching for him and giving him the treat should be minuscule, a quarter of a second perhaps. Then, start working your way up to a second, then two, three, and so on. Pursuing this systematically, you'll soon be able to wait five or ten seconds *after touching your dog* to give him his treat, until eventually you won't need a treat at all. At this point, having someone touch his sensitive area will be so strongly associated with the idea of a treat that when he sees the hand coming he will already be looking for his treat. In the hundreds of times that you will have reached for him during the course of these exercises, he will have had no bad experiences with it, and so he'll develop an enormous degree of trust and view the entire experience in a positive light.

Once your dog is totally comfortable with you and your family performing this exercise, start having friends do it with him as often as possible, too. And if you can get any kids to help out, that would be even better. In each case you may have to start at square one; but once your dog has learned to trust the entire process with one person, it will be a lot easier for him to trust the next one, and then the next one, and so on. The idea is that when the day comes that someone reaches for your dog outside the context of this exercise, he'll just assume that it's the same old game again and be totally relaxed about it.

Once you've managed to condition your dog to being touched in sensitive areas, it would be a good idea to take this one step further and begin to roughhouse with him, as described on page 37. If you'll recall, I talked about interacting with the dog in slightly annoying ways to teach him to accept childlike handling. If you can get your touch-sensitive dog to take this in stride, you've come a long way indeed.

As with the other exercises in desensitization, how long this will take depends on your dog. When fear is involved, you must be patient and work at your dog's pace rather than at the pace you might like to work. The fact is, paradoxically, the slower and more systematically you work, the faster you get results.

What If My Dog Is Emotionally Dependent and Afraid of Being Left Alone?

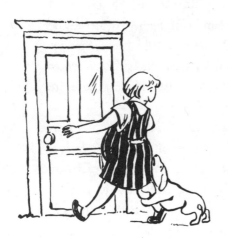

The dog who is emotionally dependent on her owner (always underfoot, can't make a move without you), or who has separation anxiety, is also the dog who potentially will have the greatest difficulty adjusting to the arrival of a child. A dog suffering from separation anxiety has difficulty tolerating being left alone, and this may result in nuisance barking, destructive behavior, or elimination in the house. The same dog may also have difficulty with the idea that she is not the center of your universe.

IS THIS NATURAL?

Of all the unnatural things we ask our dogs to do — such as heel, sit, lie down, stay, and so on — perhaps there is none more difficult than spending long periods of time alone. Dogs, like humans, are pack animals, and in a natural setting they will spend every moment of their lives surrounded by their pack members. However, to live successfully in a human world your dog must learn to spend time alone. Do her a favor and make alone time a daily part of her routine. Doing so will put her at ease and prevent innumerable difficult behavior problems.

Clearly, once your child arrives your dog will necessarily no longer be the focal point of your affections as often as she is now. In this context, it would be easy for her to interpret your child's arrival as the cause of the perceived deterioration in her relationship with you. In order to prevent this, it's important to deal with emotional neediness and separation anxiety as soon as possible before the arrival of your child, so that the necessary changes in your relationship are not associated with your baby. And, changes in the nature of your relationship are precisely what's called for. Specifically, the emotional nature of the relationship with your dog needs to be toned down, and she must be conditioned to accept increasing periods of time away from you. I understand that this may be difficult for you, but keep in mind that the attention you now shower on her will soon be flowing to your new child, potentially leaving the dog feeling left out in the cold and consequently resentful.

Even if your dog isn't especially emotionally dependent or suffering from separation anxiety, the implementation of the program outlined in the following pages, perhaps in a diluted form, is advisable anyway, since normally the arrival of a baby puts serious limitations on the amount of time a person can spend with his dog.

So the obvious question is: How do you tone down the sometimes overemotional and dependent nature of your relationship with such a dog and teach her to spend time alone? The answer, as with most things in behavior modification, is to introduce the change in small increments. If your dog tends to follow you around like a shadow, begin by having her hold down-stays for just a few moments as you go from one place to another. If she does not know the command "down-stay," you can simply tie her to something like the leg of a sofa or table (and of course you can teach her this command).

The important thing is to leave for only *a brief period of time*. How long a dog may be left varies from dog to dog, but it should be a period she can tolerate with as little stress as possible. In other words, return before she crosses her threshold of fear. For some dogs that might mean two seconds. Whatever it is, that's what you work with. When you return to your dog's vicinity, you should simply ignore her — that is, *don't look at her, don't speak to her, and don't touch her*. Just be in her space while keeping the level of your interaction to a minimum. This is what I mean when I say tone down the emotional nature of your relationship. If you constantly coddle, pet, and talk to the dog, she becomes addicted to that steady level of attention — it is precisely this addiction that you're trying to wean her away from.

Once you've returned to your dog's vicinity, you shouldn't wait too long to depart again. If your first departure lasted all of two seconds, then maybe make it three seconds this time. It all depends on your dog. Again, *be sure to return before she crosses her fear threshold*. Repeat this procedure as often as possible, slowly increasing the increments of time she can be left alone. You'll find that the amount of time it takes you to get from two seconds to five minutes will be much longer than getting from five minutes to ten minutes and so on. As the dog learns to ignore your comings and goings — because they are now so frequent — it will become easier and easier for her to tolerate increasing amounts of time alone.

If you want to make the entire affair a bit more appealing to her, try tossing her a treat or even scattering a handful of treats just before you get up and leave, but be low key about it. Simply drop them there on your way out of the area. Remember, no speaking to, touching, or looking at your dog. Just leave. Dropping treats on your way out will help your dog focus on something positive rather than on the fact that you're leaving, and help her build a positive association with your departure. And by scattering a handful across the room you will keep her busy for a while, which will dissipate the emotional intensity she normally experiences when you leave.

As you increase the periods of time that you are able to leave your dog, you can replace the treats with a favorite food-related toy *that she gets only* when you leave the area — such us a raw, frozen beef bone, a Kong Toy, or any of an assortment of "interactive dog toys" that use food inside the toy to get your dog's attention. Whatever it is, it should be something that the dog really likes and *that she gets at no other time*. And as soon as you return from your outing you should pick up the toy *and continue to ignore the dog*. This will teach her that she has access to this special item only when you're gone, and it will prevent her from getting emotionally charged up upon your return. When you use this approach, your dog will learn over time that after you leave you'll be back soon, and that she now has a window of opportunity to get something wonderful she will not get when you are around. Repeating this exercise as often as possible will help your dog develop the emotional stamina and trust that she needs in order to be left alone for increasingly long periods.

Once you've achieved some baseline success with your dog, begin leaving her in different parts of the house for longer and longer periods so that she doesn't associate alone time with just one place. Also, during the times when you're not explicitly doing these exercises, be sure to reduce how frequently you express your affection to the dog. If she's always in your lap, on the sofa next to you, or in your bed at night, begin restricting such interactions, with the goal of eliminating them almost altogether. This might sound extreme. After all, if you can't cuddle with your dog and be affectionate with her, what's the point of having her? But the purpose of this restriction is to teach her to feel emotionally secure without constantly being emotionally propped up. Once you've gotten her to the point where she can feel emotionally secure without them, you can reintroduce these interactions in measured doses and in a way that they don't create a dependency. Emotional insecurity is a terrible state to be in, so what this program calls for is the temporary sacrificing of your own emotional need to be physically close with your dog, for the sake of her mental health and well-being.

It's important, though, to keep in mind what I said a moment ago: *cut down the frequency of your displays of affection in small increments.* The idea is to reduce the frequency, not simply to cut her off. For example, if your dog has been sleeping in the bed with you for the last six years, don't start by putting her in the garage, or you're guaranteed to have a full-blown freak-out on your hands that will set your efforts back enormously. Instead, start by putting a dog

bed next to your own and tying her to the foot of your bed, so that she's got enough room to get comfy but can't jump back up and get under the covers with you. Once she's okay with that, begin scooting her bed farther and farther away from your own until she can sleep just outside your bedroom door. Similarly, if your dog is always on your lap or on the sofa next to you, begin by having her at your feet and off the sofa. Then, perhaps using the same dog bed, you can condition her to stay farther and farther away. Throughout all this, be sure to reduce the amount of petting, cooing, and general coddling as well.

Now that we have an outline, let's take a look at a few potential bumps in the road and discuss how to deal with them. The first one relates to the dog who starts whining, barking, and otherwise complaining the moment she senses she's alone. While, as I said, the goal is to return to your dog before she hits her anxiety threshold, there will be times when, despite your best efforts, your dog will resort to attention-getting behaviors almost immediately. This will likely mean that she's found in the past they worked. Now is the time for her to learn that they'll work no longer, that there is a behavior boundary you will not allow her to cross.

If your dog begins to bark, you can (a) quickly rush into the room, squirt her on the mouth and nose area with water or Bitter Apple spray, firmly tell her, "Quiet," and then immediately leave the room; or (b) rush back into the room and put her through a mind-numbing obedience drill, such as sit-down-sit-stand-down and so on, until she gets visibly bored. Demand tight compliance, and when you've pushed the dog beyond the point where she's had enough, leave the room once more. She might decide that it's better to be left with her Kong Toy than to be drilled like this by you.

Concerning the claim that negative attention is better than no attention, that your dog is still getting a payoff from your presence, even if it's unpleasant — I don't buy it. If you make your responses unpleasant enough, at some point your dog will cease and desist. However, there are a couple of other options that you can explore that don't entail going back to your dog: one is to slam your hand loudly against a nearby door, wall, or other item likely to startle the dog; the other is to loudly rattle a shake can (an empty soda can with five or six pennies in it) without saying a word. And if she resorts to chronic barking, you might consider a citronella barking collar, which is readily available online. One of these approaches will work with most dogs.

Departures and homecomings constitute another important area to consider in the resolution of separation anxiety. With respect to these, be sure to ignore your dog for ten to fifteen minutes before leaving and ten to fifteen minutes upon your return. Departures that involve a lot of interaction with your dog merely work her up emotionally, so that the moment the door closes behind you she feels she's been hung out to dry, which sends her anxiety level through the roof. Enthusiastic returns are similar because they trigger an enormous emotional spike, and they highlight for your dog the vast emotional difference between when you're there and when you're not. Of course, the whole idea is to narrow the qualitative difference between when you're there and when you're not, in order to help relieve your dog of the wild emotional swings that trigger attacks of anxiety.

To further alleviate your dog's distress at your departures, it is helpful to teach her to ignore predeparture cues. Most dogs are acutely aware of the patterns leading up to your departure — they see you pulling your coat from the closet, slipping on your shoes, jingling your keys, and so on. These events can trigger anxiety attacks, so reducing their relevance to your dog, as well as ignoring her before your departure, can be helpful. As with many of the exercises described so far, this one is simple but sometimes tedious. The trick is to go through your predeparture routine as often as possible, without actually leaving. For example, pick up and jingle your keys and then set them down again. March over to the closet and pull out your coat, only to hang it up again. Of course, totally ignore the dog throughout all this. And as often as possible string all these events together in the sequence that you follow when you actually leave; and if you can do this at the same times of day that you normally leave, so much the better. The more often you do this, the quicker it will dissolve your dog's anxiety over your departures.

A related issue that often arises with needy dogs is jealousy. For instance, it's not uncommon for a dog to become annoyed and intrusive upon seeing two members of the household engaged in displays of affection such as hugs. Some dogs will even bark, try to push themselves between the owners, or pursue an array of other attention-getting behaviors that will bring the affectionate displays to an end. I've even had clients whose dogs threw fits when they talked on the phone. The problems in relation to raising a child under these circumstances should be obvious. Teach your dog that such interruptions are unacceptable, and help her build a new and positive association with affectionate displays between household members.

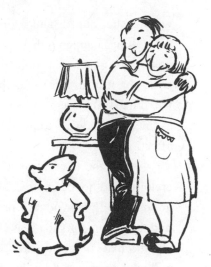

There'll be none of that…

Begin by setting up as many displays of affection as possible (this is the fun part) and then reprimanding your dog for any intrusions. My definition of an intrusion is encroaching within five feet of where the affection is taking place and then barking or engaging in anything else intrusive and annoying. My favorite response, once again, is the trusty squirt bottle filled with either water or Bitter Apple spray. A Pet Corrector should also do the trick. If your dog gets too close, then, in a firm tone, give her the command "out" and squirt her on the nose and mouth or startle her with compressed air. For most dogs, this sudden shock will provide ample pause for reflection. A few repetitions and you'll likely see the behavior subside.

Of course, as with almost everything else in behavior modification, you want to couple a positive alternative with any form of reprimand. So, once you've managed to halt your dog's annoying interruptions, you can take the corresponding step of teaching her to look forward to your displays of affection by helping her build positive associations with them. Simply arrange it so that, just as the staged affections begin, she gets a favorite bone, toy, or treat to chew on. And in order to round off the association and drive it home, remove the yummy items from your dog when the affectionate displays are over. This will help her quickly and strongly associate the two events and teach her that good things happen to her when others display affection. And notably, those good things happen at some distance from you, building increasing comfort with physical distance into the interaction. As her views begin to change, you'll need to do less and less of this, and your dog, formerly seeing herself as jilted, will now be content without inserting herself into the midst of your affections.

In addition to everything discussed so far, the primary importance of exercise should not be ignored. I have already affirmed the adage "Tired dogs are good dogs." If your dog is a pressure cooker of pent-up energy that she hasn't had the opportunity to release, it should come as no surprise that she will easily channel that energy into her anxiety. On the other hand, if she is exhausted she will have correspondingly less energy available to fuel her fear. Energy is easily translated into anxiety, and exhaustion is more readily translated into sleep. Sleeping dogs don't worry about the whereabouts of their owners. They dream dog dreams and so are otherwise occupied. This means that working with your dog in the routines outlined here is going to be much more effective when your dog has had ample exercise and physical exhaustion.

Finally, some dogs, despite their owners' best efforts, are so deeply anxious that they are virtually impossible to rehabilitate with conventional methods of behavior modification such as the ones highlighted here. It seems that no matter how much work you do with a dog like that, the results are never better than marginal. In such cases it might be advisable to consider antianxiety medications, which can provide a bridge and allow you to gain a foothold in the resolution of the dog's fear. They can create receptivity on the part of your dog that simply was not there before. With this opening, the effects of your exercises will be radically improved.

But note that the antianxiety medications, at least in the way that I view them, are not a solution in themselves. They are simply an aid to the routines

I've outlined. If through the use of such medications you can get your dog to relax enough to consider the new habits and associations built by these training exercises, then, after the dog has had sufficient exposure to the exercises, you should be able to wean her off the medications. The exercises will have created new learned behaviors and associations that, hopefully, will stick once the dog is taken off the medications.

JUST SAY MAYBE!

The following medications are effective at relieving anxiety, and new ones are coming out all the time. Speak to your veterinarian to learn which of them might be appropriate for your dog, and never use any medication without the advice of a vet. In other words, please don't share your Prozac. Also, see note 1 in this chapter.

- Elavil (amitriptyline)
- Prozac (fluoxetine)
- Xanax (alprazolam)

How long medication takes to ease anxiety can be hard to predict, but I usually advise my clients to prepare for six months of work when attempting to resolve issues involving extreme emotional dependency and separation anxiety. That is not to say things can't be resolved sooner; I mention it simply to prepare you psychologically for the possibility that they might not be and to help you resolve to keep trying. With respect to medications, since new ones are coming out all the time and will be available only by prescription, you should speak with your veterinarian about them. If your vet is not that knowledgeable about these substances, ask him or her to recommend someone who is.[1]

DOG-APPEASING PHEROMONES

In addition to pharmaceutical-strength antianxiety medications, you might try dog-appeasing pheromones (they can easily be used in conjunction with pharmaceutical meds), sold under the name Adaptil (formerly DAP). A synthetic version of a dog pheromone produced by lactating females, it has been shown to relax anxious dogs. It comes in the form of a plug-in diffuser, collar, or spray, all of which are readily available online.

Let's take a moment to summarize the program in simple terms. Begin by toning down the overemotional nature of the relationship you have with your dog. Do this using the exercises described here, but be sure to implement them in increments your dog can handle. Simply cutting your dog off from affection can actually kick her into a full-blown anxiety attack and set your efforts back enormously! Remember the tortoise and the hare: slow but steady wins the race. Help your dog build new, better associations with what it means to be alone, by providing positive experiences to occupy her in your absence. Also, do what you reasonably can to exercise and tire your dog. If necessary, investigate the use of antianxiety medications to make inroads into your dog's anxiety issues. Finally, give yourself as much time as possible to make this work. Don't start with these exercises two weeks before your baby is due or, worse, after your baby's arrival. By then it may be too late. Start now![2]

What If My Dog Is Possessive of Toys or Food?

Object and food guarding is perhaps one of the most common and most dangerous issues you face when bringing dogs and children together. Since dogs often view children as lower-ranking pack members and potential competitors for valued resources, the likelihood of trouble should be taken especially seriously. If your dog has bitten or threatened to bite you in this context, please read the section "Dealing with a Dangerous Dog," on page 92. If your dog gets tense around objects or food but has not bitten or threatened to, then read on.

To begin with, if your dog exhibits signs of object guarding, be sure that you've assertively implemented the Doggie Twelve-Step Program described in

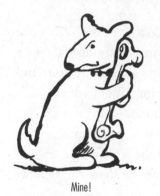

Mine!

chapter 1. After all, if your dog is guarding objects against you, the first question you should ask yourself is why he feels he has the right to do this. Since he clearly doesn't respect you as leader, that's the obvious place to start. Once you've successfully implemented the program and established a foundation of respect, proceed with the routines outlined in the following pages, which teach your dog to both trust you and expect something positive as you approach

him when he's near his food and favorite objects. By way of example, I'll share a story.

A long time ago a beautiful and sweet ten-month-old Rottweiler named Otis stayed at my home for two weeks of boarding and training while his parents set off on a European vacation. I had known Otis since he was about eight weeks old, and you couldn't want a sweeter dog. There wasn't a mean bone in his body, and he was completely tolerant of anything the three small children in his household could dish out. So imagine my surprise, on Otis's first night at my home, when I walked near him while he was eating and he began growling at me. I was shocked.

After reprimanding him I immediately phoned the owners, hoping to catch them before they left on their trip and talk to them about this. The first thing I asked was if they fed Otis alone in an isolated area. I knew the answer would be yes, and indeed it was. When I informed the owner of what happened, he responded with surprise: "Well, he's never done that before." Of course he hadn't. Nobody had ever come near him while he was eating. Otis always got to eat alone in the garage, and everyone was instructed not to disturb him. "What are you going to do if one of your kids accidentally goes near him while he's eating?" I asked. "Uh, well, I guess I don't know," came the reply.

Clearly, growling at you while eating or in relation to any other high-value object is unacceptable behavior; and from the moment you realize there's a problem, you should work to ensure that your dog will never be protective or aggressive around food or toys of any kind. The implications of this with respect to the new child in your life should be obvious.

If you're not sure how your dog will react, now would be a good time to test him. Go near him and simply stand there while he is chewing a favorite bone or eating his meal, and see what he does. Does he show any signs of discomfort or unease? Displays of discomfort, in the case of meals, most commonly take one of two forms: Suddenly eating rapidly, with an intensity that he usually doesn't exhibit, as if he wants to gobble everything down before you have a chance to take it. Or conversely, suddenly getting tense and eating exceedingly slowly with a paranoid look on his face. In the case of favorite bones and toys, he might express either of those attitudes or simply feel the need to take his toy or bone to some special place and chew it while on his own, jealously protecting it like Gollum guarding his ring.

If you find yourself with issues along these lines, then implement the following routine. Let's begin with the food bowl. If your dog exhibits tension as you approach him during a meal, begin by walking near him while he's eating, but not close enough to elicit a reaction. As you pass him, throw a treat in his direction and keep going. After he picks it up and goes back to his dish, repeat the procedure. Keep doing this until your dog anticipates that you're going to throw him a treat each time you enter his "zone," and then slowly begin moving closer to him. Still, only *pass through* his zone — that is, walk by, toss him the treat, and keep walking. This way he will not feel that you are truly encroaching on his zone. You're just passing through and leaving a goodie in your wake. That's not so bad. You'll notice that soon, as you approach, your dog will lift his head from his bowl in anticipation of the treat. When this happens, it's time to start moving a little closer to him, and then a little closer, and so on. Eventually you'll be standing right next to him tossing treats into or near his dish (depends on your aim) while he's eating.

Now it's time to start touching him during his meal. Gently place your hand on his back or side as he's eating; and while you're touching him, throw treats into his dish. In the beginning, you might have to throw treats in relatively rapid succession, but as your dog gets habituated to this you can continually slow down the treat count. Eventually, your dog will have no problem with you standing near him and touching him while he's having his meal. As long as things are moving along well, continue by touching the dog in an increasingly pronounced manner. While initially you might have only rested your hand on his back, you should graduate to stroking him across increasingly larger areas of his body for longer and longer periods of time. When you've arrived at this point, your dog should have no problem with you standing near him and touching him while he's eating. He will no longer be protective of his zone. Once you can do this, have other members of the household practice as well, until your dog is no longer distressed when people stand near him as he eats.

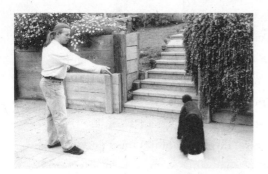

From outside your dog's reaction zone, toss her a treat while she's eating.

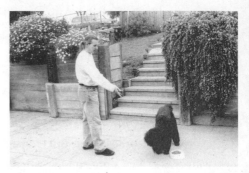

As she gets more comfortable with this, move closer. Take your time and don't rush it.

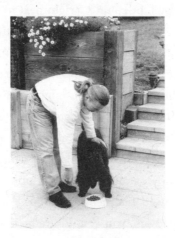

Continue until you can stand next to her and touch her while dropping treats in the dish.

Keep in mind that in real life, getting from the first of these photos to the third could take a few weeks.

This brings you to the next exercise: actually taking the bowl away from the dog. There are two approaches you can use here, and which one you choose will be a field decision you'll have to make based on your intuition and observations. If you feel that you can safely reach in and grab your dog's dish without creating a response, go ahead and do so. Quickly place a yummy treat (like cheese or chicken or meat — something he never sees at any other time) on top of the dog's food and *immediately* return it to him. The key word here is *immediately*. Make this quick, and don't give him obedience commands. This is not about showing him who's boss. It's about building trust.

If you don't feel good about this, you'll have to start at a more basic level. Sit on the floor with two bowls in your possession: an empty one, and one with his meal in it. With the bowls on one side of you and your dog on the other, take a handful of food out of the full dish, place it in the empty one, and hold it in front of your dog. *Do not let go of the dish!* Continue to hold on to it while the dog is eating, and when he's through pull the dish away and place another handful of food in it. Then, repeat the procedure. This will get your dog used to the idea that your hand is near his dish often, and that when your hand removes his dish it will momentarily return it with more food. In other words, your removal of the dish is a prelude to more food, not to losing a valued resource.

When you've arrived at this point, you are ready for the next step. Put several handfuls of food in your dog's dish, and then take it away from him before he's finished, placing a delicious treat on top of it and promptly returning it to him. Let him empty the bowl, and then repeat this procedure until he is totally comfortable with it. Only when your dog is habituated to this routine and has no problem with it should you take your hand off the food dish — just momentarily. Then reach in again and repeat the procedure. Gradually increase the time you leave your hand off the dish before reaching in to take it again. By the time you get to this point, your dog will have watched you take

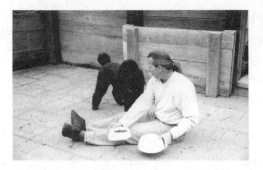

1. Have an empty and full dish on one side of you and your dog on the other.

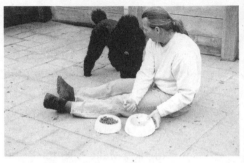

2. Put a handful of kibble in the empty bowl and...

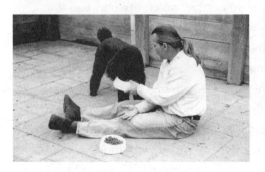

3. ...give it to the dog.

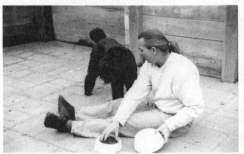

4. Repeat this process until the meal is done.

his dish away so many times that it simply won't matter to him anymore. This, of course, is the whole idea. Once you're at this juncture, you can bring the two elements of this program together. That is, approach your dog while he's eating, take his dish up, place a treat on top, and return it to him. Then, leave the area. A few minutes later repeat the procedure, and soon your dog will be comfortable with having you around his food dish.

Once everything looks okay, you should add a third element: the "off" command. If you're not sure how to teach this command, refer to the section

"Do Not Let the Dog Take Food without Your Permission," on page 29, step 9 in the Doggie Twelve-Step Program. If you've done everything right so far, then when you walk up to your dog's dish while he's eating, and you issue the command "off," he should take several steps back from his dish. Then you can pick it up, place several delicious treats in it, and return it to him. Practice this once or twice per mealtime until your dog has internalized this routine. And once your dog is comfortable with all this, be sure to have everyone in the household try it. Of course, the point is to teach him to trust you and anticipate something wonderful when you approach the food dish. This will undermine the need he feels to defend his area and so will resolve his resource-guarding issues.

Finally, from here on out, do not allow your dog to stake out his own private eating zones around your house. Feed him in the busiest places at the busiest times of the day so that he gets used to being surrounded by plenty of commotion during mealtimes and, in this way, relinquishes his need for privacy.

So far, the object-guarding issues we have discussed have been related only to the food dish. What about toys, bones, and other high-value objects? If your dog is possessive about any of these things, you'll have to implement a similar routine. Let's quickly apply to this new situation the lessons learned so far. If you've been following the Doggie Twelve-Step Program, you will by now have restricted your dog's access to toys and objects he considered his own (see step 9 of the Doggie Twelve-Step Program). What follows is a great exercise to reintroduce these valued objects.

Begin by taking something the dog really loves, like a big fat knuckle bone, sit down on the floor, and hand it to him. However, *do not let it go*. Hold on to one end while your dog is chewing on it so that he never has the full sense of possessing it. Once he's chewed on it for a little while, give the command "off" (see step 8 of the Doggie Twelve-Step Program), pull the bone away, give him a treat, and hand the bone back to him — while still holding on to it — so he can continue to chew on it. After a few more moments repeat the procedure. Each time, let the dog gnaw on the bone a little bit longer than the time before, allowing him to get increasingly into it. Again and again, issue the command "off," take it away, give him a treat, and return the bone. Keep in mind that, for the moment, *you should not take your hand off the bone.* This prevents your dog from feeling a full sense of ownership and allows you to teach him what will happen if he releases it: he gets a treat and then gets his bone back. From your dog's standpoint this could be viewed as "doggie in-

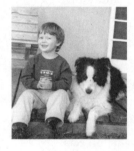

Photo: Mike Wombacher

vesting": give up the principal (his bone) for a brief period of time, receive the interest (the treat), and then get the principal back. All in all, a good deal.

Once your dog is comfortable with this routine, you can go to the next step. Again allow your dog to chew on the bone while you hold one end. However, this time let go of the bone for just a moment or two, then grab it again, issue the command "off," give him a treat, and return the bone just as you did before. The only difference is that now you're taking your hand off the bone for a moment: for a short time, your dog has full possession of it. And we want to increase the length of that time in steady increments. In other words, leave your hand off the bone for a bit longer, and then longer, and longer, until you can leave your hand off the bone for as long as you like before reaching in, taking it, giving him a treat, returning it, and so on.

When this is going well, it's time to add the last couple of steps. Give your dog his bone, get up and walk away, return a few moments later, bend down, have him release it, and once again give him a treat before returning it. When your dog is comfortable with that, the final step involves simply approaching him while he's chewing on his bone, issuing the command "off" before reaching in to get the bone, bending over to pick it up, giving him a treat, and returning the bone. Once you're at this point, have everyone in your household try it, and soon your dog will be trustworthy around objects. And finally, bear in mind that you literally cannot practice these exercises too often, and that the more iterations of these exercises your dog experiences over a short time frame the better.

Now, you might be wondering why I don't simply recommend a straight punitive approach, like a yank on a training collar or even a correction with an electronic collar, whenever your dog gives you trouble around objects he considers his own. The primary reason is that this might work if *you* are taking the object from the dog, since you're the one dishing out the punishment, but your dog will not have the same level of respect for your young child. So, while he might tolerate this treatment from you, he most likely will not from a baby, who, as I've said, he'll tend to view as a lower-ranking pack member. Moreover, an approach using strictly force will tend to confirm the dog's worst suspicions: the presence of people around his food dish is bad news.

When you follow the program outlined here, your dog will learn to trust you and others around his food dish, and so his initial motivation for guarding it will be undermined. He will have learned that most of the time he not only gets his object back, but he gets a treat to boot. Even when you're no longer using treats in this context, your dog will have become so conditioned to the new routine that the old problem simply won't show up anymore. This is not to say that force used in conjunction with the approaches outlined here is never appropriate — it might be. However, it should be considered primarily as a last resort and used while you are working in conjunction with a professional trainer who is familiar with all that has been laid out here.

What If My Dog Barks Excessively?

If your dog is a nuisance barker, that in itself is so annoying that it warrants being dealt with. But when you have a newborn in the house, dealing with the barker will quickly become a top priority. After all, during the early stages of parenthood the level of sleep deprivation is notorious. Add a sporadically barking dog who will startle you and your child out of precious moments of sleep, and you'll have a frustrating situation on your hands in no time. It's important that any barking problem be handled long before your child arrives, since once the baby's born you may not have the patience or energy to work with your dog.

Before starting, let's note that barking is a perfectly natural doggie behavior, and that the elimination of all barking is neither feasible nor sensible. You should, however, be able to limit your dog's barking to appropriate times and places, when it won't create a problem for anyone. Any number of situations will cause your dog to bark, but whatever the case you have two ways to respond. The first is to teach the dog the "quiet" command, and the second is to use a barking collar. Which you choose depends on your situation, and often people use both.

Teaching the dog the "quiet" command is a simple and straightforward affair. Take a squirt bottle that has a fairly powerful and direct stream, and fill it with either water or a taste deterrent like Bitter Apple (for some dogs, shake cans and Pet Correctors work better). Have this with you whenever possible. This will enable you to reprimand your dog the moment she starts barking, and you won't have to go looking for the bottle at key moments. If your dog predictably barks only in certain locations, such as the front door or window, permanently place the bottle, shake can, or Pet Corrector there for easy access.

When your dog begins to bark and you've had enough, simply go up to her and issue the command "quiet," wait a moment, and then squirt her right on the nose and mouth if she doesn't stop. *It's important to wait a moment between the bark and the squirt so that the dog has the opportunity to comply.* Of course, in the beginning she won't know what "quiet" means, so inevitably she'll get squirted; but as time goes on, she'll learn to identify the word *quiet* as a warning and respond with silence. If your dog resumes barking within the next minute or so, then you may simply squirt her at the same moment that you say "quiet," since at this point it's a reprimand rather than an instruction. You want her to understand that once you say "quiet" it means she should stop barking for a while, not simply offer you three seconds of silence.

Be as sneaky as a ninja with your bottle, pulling it from behind your back or out of your pocket for just a second, squirting your dog, and then quickly hiding it from her view. You don't want her to learn that "quiet" has meaning only when you've got a bottle around. Let her believe that you potentially have it on you at all times. You want her to learn that the key variable here is the word *quiet* and not the squirt bottle. If your crafty dog quickly figures out that your bottle's range is limited, I recommend letting her drag a leash around the house for a few days while you're working on this. That way, if she attempts to make a run for it, you can simply step on the leash and still reprimand her. Crude but effective![3]

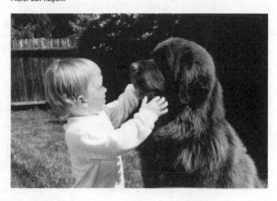

Photo: Bari Halperin

This is the basic routine for establishing the word *quiet* as part of your dog's vocabulary. Now, let's take a quick look at a few permutations of this exercise that should help you meet the needs of a variety of situations. One thing you eventually want your dog to learn is to obey your "quiet" command from a distance. You don't want her to keep barking until you can get to her and threaten her with a squirt from the bottle or a blast from the Pet Corrector. The key is to teach your dog that she gets only one opportunity to refrain from barking before something unpleasant happens. In the beginning, if you hear your dog barking on the other side of the house, *don't say a word*. Let her bark, but begin rapidly moving in her direction. Only when you are within bottle or Pet Corrector range do you issue the command "quiet," just once. Then you squirt her or blast her with air. Doing this will teach your dog to pay attention to your commands even when you're not right next to her — that is, it will begin to condition her to respond to "quiet" the first time around.

Once this is accomplished you can take the next step. Follow exactly the same routine, but this time issue your command from several feet farther out. If your dog bursts out with another bark, leap to her side and squirt or blast her. Once she's responsive from the new distance, move farther away in increments until you find that your dog responds to the "quiet" command from anywhere in the house. Should she decide to test you at some point (most dogs will) by continuing to bark when you're at a distance, then immediately tell her "no" repeatedly and in a commanding tone as you run to where she's barking, and then correct her. Continuing to issue the reprimand "no" until you reach her ties the squirt or air blast she gets from you back to the beginning of her infraction and allows you to reprimand her after the fact.

If your dog is one of those crafty characters who keeps barking until you appear, and then suddenly quiets down, squirt her anyway. Teach her that once she's blown off your initial "quiet" command, it's too late, she's doomed. A squirt or air blast is unavoidable. Using this approach, you'll soon have a dog who responds to your "quiet" command appropriately: with silence. What successfully implementing such a routine means is that, in any situation, you can choose whether to allow your dog to bark or not. This is important, because there will be circumstances when you want your dog to bark, such as when a stranger comes to the door.

Of course there may be times when you are in neither the mood nor the position to command your dog to be quiet. For instance, if your baby has just fallen asleep, telling your dog to be quiet after she has already started barking would be nearly pointless, since the damage is done: both you and your child are now awake. For situations like this and others where you simply want your dog to be quiet without any instruction from you, I recommend barking collars. There are two effective varieties: citronella spray collars and electronic collars (ultrasonic collars that emit annoying sounds, which only your dog can hear, are also available, but in my experience they are ineffective). I prefer the citronella spray collar, because it is pain free and utterly harmless. It simply sprays your dog under the muzzle with citronella spray, derived from a citrus-based essential oil, which smells good to humans and apparently horrible to dogs. Your dog barks, she gets sprayed. It's that simple. It's annoying but pain free, the timing is perfect every time, and you don't have to be there. Your dog quickly learns that when she has the collar on, barking is unacceptable; in relatively short order she'll maintain silence when wearing the collar. End of problem! If you want to take a nap with your baby, fit your dog with the collar and go to sleep.

For about 85 percent of dogs, citronella collars are supremely effective. However, there are hard cases who will either be unaffected by the collar or figure out that if they bark about fifteen to twenty times they will empty the collar and then they're home free. For these dogs I recommend electronic collars. Some people might find this harsh, but I assure you that your dog will not be getting corrected very often. It's unfortunate but true that pain, even the momentary pain caused by such a collar, is a powerful motivator. Your dog will quickly learn that wearing the collar demands silence, and after learning this she will soon decide to stop testing the collar. The number of corrections from an electronic collar that a dog will experience is usually quite low.[4] If you want to buy an electronic collar, I recommend seeking the assistance of a professional trainer and finding a collar that allows you to set the stimulation level according to the sensitivity of your dog. That way you can find the level that's just enough to get the job done and can minimize the discomfort she has to experience while learning to be silent.

The good news about barking collars is that you may not have to use one for long — perhaps only six to eight weeks, and perhaps far less. That's because your dog will likely learn to identify a particular situation with the demand for silence. This is called *situational learning.* Consider the following

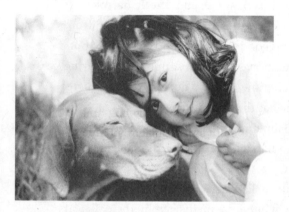

Photo: Candyce Plummer Gaudiani Photography

example. One of the peculiarities of my own life at one point was that I ran a meditation center at my home. This meant that between 7:30 and 8:30 every evening I needed total silence in the house. At that time I had an enthusiastic and high-energy standard poodle who loved people and would bark exuberantly whenever anyone came to the house. Realizing I had a problem, I put a citronella collar on her and, predict-

ably, the barking evaporated. Interestingly, I found that after about a month of wearing the collar she no longer needed it. She'd learned that this particular circumstance demanded silence, and she simply became conditioned to it. I never had another barking problem with her.

It can also be helpful to teach your dog a new set of responses to certain stimuli that cause barking. You can do this by building new and positive associations with them for the dog, which in turn will lead to responses incompatible with barking. Consider the following. The classic example of a conditioned barking response is found in the dog who always barks at the sound of the doorbell. Wouldn't it be nice if, when your dog heard the doorbell ring, instead of running to the door barking like crazy she ran to you and sat at your feet with rapt attention? Training your dog to do this is easier than you think.

Some years ago I had a client with one of the most resolute chronic barkers I'd ever met — a miniature Dachshund — who taught her dog to do this in about a week and a half. She began by having someone stand outside her door and ring the bell as my client stood on the inside armed with a squirt bottle and sprayed her dog each time he barked. She was teaching him: "No barking at the door, period." It took her some time to totally squelch the bark response, since it was so powerfully conditioned in her dog that he literally could not help himself. But eventually he made the choice not to bark. *That's when she immediately rewarded him with a treat.* Soon he learned that if he barked he got sprayed and if he didn't he got a reward — a perfect example of how positives and negatives work powerfully together. From that point on the momentum of his conditioning changed and he quickly learned to respond to the doorbell by being quiet and receiving a treat.

Getting to this point with a dog on a consistent basis may take a few days, but it will definitely happen. You can accelerate this process by recording about a minute's worth of doorbell rings and playing them back to your dog throughout the day. Each time she hears the recorded bell ring, guess what? She gets a treat. Once she's figured this out, try playing the recorded ring with the dog at some distance from you. When she hears it, encourage her to come to you to get her treat. In due course you'll find that when she hears the doorbell ring, she will come to you for her treat rather than rushing the door in a barking frenzy — a total turnabout in her behavior.

I have a couple of final observations about barking. Sometimes the best solutions are the easiest ones, and so they are overlooked. For instance, if your dog barks because she's running around in the backyard chasing cats or squirrels, or she's hanging around the front window going off at every passerby, the simplest solution might be to deny her access to these areas. When you need some silence, perhaps she should be in her crate or a quiet part of the house chewing on a favorite bone. Also, be aware that barking is often a boredom-related behavior. Your dog might be barking simply because there isn't anything else to do and, let's face it, barking is fun. Giving your dog more exercise and playtime, after which she will come home exhausted, would be especially helpful. Once again, tired dogs are good dogs.

At any rate, an intelligent combination of the suggestions outlined here should help you eliminate any barking problems long before your child arrives. And of course, finding a solution to those problems will give you peace of mind and allow you to spend your energy where you should: caring for your baby.

What If My Dog Is Overprotective?

If your dog is overprotective of you, it's highly likely that he'll express the same behavior in relation to your child. For example, he may inappropriately "protect" your child against someone who has every right to be there, such as a friend or a babysitter. If your dog has bitten or threatened to bite in this context, please read the section "Dealing with a Dangerous Dog," on page 92. If you feel that your dog has the potential to become a problem, read on.

TOO MUCH OF A GOOD THING

While we all would like our dogs to feel protective of us, it can be a mixed blessing. Be sure your dog feels responsible *to you* rather than *for you*. A dog who feels responsible to you will look to you for guidance and direction in all things. That means you'll be able to help him make decisions. A dog who feels responsible for you will make his own decisions, decisions that are usually inappropriate and sometimes dangerous.

The first thing to do with a dog like this is to be sure you are fully implementing the Doggie Twelve-Step Program, outlined in chapter 1 (see page 5).

This is particularly important in the case of overprotective dogs, because they are almost always confused about their status in their pack. Part of the pack leader's job is to protect pack members; and if your dog mistakenly believes that leadership is part of his job description, he is likely to make some serious errors of judgment in the name of protecting his pack. The difference between a dog feeling responsible *for* his owners and feeling responsible *to* his owners is critical. And when a dog is put through an effective rank-management program and learns to feel responsible to the family rather than for it, his inappropriate outbursts of aggression are likely to simply cease or be significantly diminished. If neither happens, then it's usually a relatively simple matter to make the outbursts disappear.

You can begin by keeping your dog on a leash with you or on a tie-down (essentially any means by which you can tether your dog to something — a leash around a table leg, for instance), which restricts his ability to control his perimeter and act out inappropriately outside your zone of influence. If he begins to act out by lunging or barking, simply squirt him with the Bitter Apple spray, rattle a shake can, blast a Pet Corrector, or give him a correction on his training collar. It is important for him to know that you, his leader, seriously disapprove of this behavior. Once he's inhibiting himself, redirect his energy and attention by giving him obedience commands. This shouldn't pose a problem, since theoretically you've already trained him, or are in the process of training him, to comply with the commands in the context of the rank-management program.

Once your dog is somewhat controlled — that is, *no longer fully reactive* — have some friends of yours pose as intruders and begin tossing treats to him from a safe zone, an area where there's no chance your dog can get to your friends. Additionally, instruct your "intruders" not to attempt to solicit any interactions from your dog by talking to him in a sweet tone or attempting to pet him, because this can make him apprehensive and trigger more reactivity.

Just have them continue to throw treats to him so long as he's behaving and to otherwise ignore him. Of course, if it appears that your dog would like to seek out an interaction with your guests, then by all means let him. But continue to instruct your guests to be relatively aloof and to physically engage with your dog only to the degree that he is willing to entertain such an engagement.

Repeating this procedure as often as possible, and in as many different contexts as possible, will change your dog's response to these situations. Eventually he will come to understand that anyone you allow into your home, or otherwise near you, should not only be okay with him but also could be the source of something nice.

To fully implement this change of heart, especially if your dog has been suspicious for a long time, may take a while, and there may be ups and downs. But as with everything else, if you start as soon as possible and work as diligently as possible, you should be able to overcome this problem — and probably within three to six weeks.

What If I Have More than One Dog and They Don't Get Along Well Together?

In behavioral lingo this is called *sibling rivalry*. If your dogs are experiencing a great deal of tension in relation to one another, you should consider this *a major red flag*, since many dogs tend to view children as lower-ranking pack members and potentially will treat them poorly, too. If your dogs have bitten, or threatened to bite, each other or you in this context, please read the section "Dealing with a Dangerous Dog," on page 92.

If your dogs are simply tense, moody, or jealous around one another, there are a few things you can do to straighten out the situation. First, implement the rank-management program outlined earlier and *ensure that all of your dogs unequivocally view you as their leader*. As pack leader you have the right to control conflict in your group, a right you may have to exercise. Also, assess which of your dogs is the higher-ranking one. If you're not sure, ask yourself questions such as: Does one dog occasionally prevent the other from entering the room? Does one dog habitually demand that the other get out of his way? Does one dog proudly parade a toy around in front of the other, taunting him with it but refusing to let him get it? Which dog goes out the door first if both have an equal opportunity? With a simple look and some posturing, can one dog force the other to leave the room or drop a toy? Closely observing the relationship between your dogs should help you figure out their rank.

Once you have figured this out, you must be sure to reinforce the higher-ranking dog in his position and simultaneously remind the lower-ranking dog of his subordinate status. *Failing to do so is a leading cause of serious trouble between dogs in the same home.* Dogs have a host of behaviors they display in relation to one another (such as those implied by the questions just mentioned), and they use them to peaceably work out their relationship. But in many cases the owner enters the picture and unknowingly sends the dogs signals that imply the exact opposite of what they've worked out. The most common reason for this is that people feel sorry for the underdog and start giving him special treatment. This, of course, totally annoys the naturally more dominant dog, who will be sure to go out of his way to put the other one in his place the first opportunity he gets. Having a situation like this can build unresolved tension between the dogs that can explode into cases of extreme and even deadly aggression.

Dogs who relate to each other this way will quite possibly relate to your child in the same manner. So, it's extremely important that, once you figure out who's higher ranking, you reinforce the positions they've worked out. This means that you actually treat the dominant dog preferentially *in such a way that both dogs know it*, by giving him a little more affection, better treats, more desirable resting places, and so on. Moreover, you must also reprimand the lower-ranking dog for any dominant overtures toward the higher-ranking dog. Implementing this standard, challenging as it may be to our egalitarian sensibilities, ensures that all the social signals flowing to the dogs from all aspects of their environment are consistent with what they've worked out. In this way no tension should develop between them, and there will be nothing for them to fight over. And in the event that there is tension here and there, you, as the pack leader, have the right to control social interactions in your group if needed. Remember, while in the human world equality might produce justice, in the canine world equality produces violence. Be sure to be the leader of your pack, and then understand and enforce its hierarchy.

What If My Dog Has Killed or Seriously Injured Domestic Animals?

If your dog kills domestic animals, whether yours or other people's, this is a major red flag. Usually such behavior is driven by predatory instincts and is extremely difficult to resolve *reliably*. Because of the level of force involved in the killing, having such a dog around a small child is an extremely questionable undertaking. Children have shrill, high-pitched voices and move in erratic and unpredictable ways. These are just the kind of actions that can trigger predatory responses in a dog. Each year, numerous fatalities of small children as a result of dog attacks are reported. A great many of those are perpetrated by the family dog, and often prey motivation is the culprit. In a number of cases the dog actually went up to the infant's crib, pulled it out, and killed it. If you have a dog who has killed or seriously injured a domestic animal, I strongly recommend finding a new home for the dog as soon as possible. For more on this, please read the section in this chapter titled "Dealing with a Dangerous Dog."

In closing my discussion of specific problem behaviors, I should highlight the fact that it takes time to resolve them; so the sooner you start working on any issues you have with your dog, the better. But even if it's rather late in the day and your baby is due anytime, or if you have already had it, there may still be time. A great many of the issues discussed here don't become real problems until your child is about eight months old. It's at this age that most kids begin crawling, and then the encounters between your dog and your child are guaranteed to be more frequent and less predictable. When your child starts walking — at about a year and two months — the frequency of their meetings will increase, and the unpredictability of these meetings will be amplified dramatically. During their interactions you'll find out whether you've done the work you need to, so please use your time wisely before that day!

TIRED DOGS ARE GOOD DOGS!

I've said it a few times throughout this book, and I'm saying it again because of its extreme importance: an overwhelming percentage of behavior problems in dogs could be eliminated or at least significantly diminished with adequate exercise. So much of what creates problems for people with their dogs is simply boredom. If you're not in a position to give your dog the exercise he needs, find someone who can. An entire industry of pet care professionals has evolved in the last few decades to help you with precisely this issue. Also, ten or fifteen minutes of tight obedience routines that your dog finds challenging and stimulating can be the equivalent of at least the same amount of time spent exercising. Whatever amount of energy you can drain out of your dog through exercise will be energy that isn't available for getting himself into trouble. So do both yourself and him a favor and give him a workout.

Dealing with a Dangerous Dog

At several points in the book so far I've directed you to read this section if your dog has actually bitten, or come close to biting, a person. This is not because the behavior modification routines I've outlined won't work for such dogs — they will — but because, when a child is involved, cases involving the possibility of real aggression need special consideration.

The main consideration, of course, is whether it's appropriate to have such a dog in the presence of a child. Assessing this question is more art than science, but there are four factors I usually consider when someone approaches me with that question: threshold of reactivity, level of intensity, previous history, and the crossover considerations.

By *threshold of reactivity*, I mean: How much of a certain type of stimulation is necessary in order to make the dog reactive (that is, act out in ways that are undesirable)? By *level of intensity*, I mean: Once the threshold of reactivity is crossed, how intense is the response? Does it involve only a bark and an effort to retreat, or does the dog lash out aggressively, including by biting? If there is biting, how severe is it? Is it a nip with the front of the mouth or a full bite with the middle or back of the mouth? Then there's *previous history*. How long is your dog's history for this kind of behavior? What kind of rap sheet does he have? Of course, the longer the history, the more powerful the momentum behind the behavior and, as a result, the greater the cause for concern.

Finally, there are *crossover considerations*. Let's say your dog is possessive of the food dish but has never done more than issue a slight growl when you approach him. Maybe not such a big deal. But what if he's also been in dogfights where he's seriously injured another dog? I would consider this a huge red flag because, though the dog's reactivity and level of intensity around the food dish is moderate, his level of intensity in relation to another dog is high. My concern would be that your dog might view your child as a competitor or lower-ranking pack member and use the same level of intensity that he previously used against other dogs. This means he would present a serious threat.

If your dog is having behavior problems that potentially involve a severely aggressive response, you should consider whether you can responsibly keep this dog in the presence of a new child. Most such problems are totally reversible and manageable, and if a child weren't involved I would most definitely argue for working with the dog. However, with a child the risks are too great (for both child and dog — for if your dog ends up biting your child, you're going to be faced with not only potentially serious injuries but also some tough choices about the life of your dog and, possibly, a legal nightmare). In cases like this, I strongly suggest finding your dog a new home.

But if you feel strongly about keeping such a dog, my advice is to immediately seek the help of a skillful behavior professional. Finding such a person can be difficult, but there are a few things to look for. Ask for recommendations at the veterinary offices in your area. Also, ask at the dog park and in your neighborhood. If the same name comes up again and again, this is a person you might check with. I suggest avoiding trainers whose primary solution to every behavior problem is a yank on a choke chain. Such a one-dimensional and strictly compulsive approach is a clear indication that this person is not really familiar with serious behavior issues. I'm not suggesting that you avoid trainers who use compulsive methods, for sometimes, when intelligently applied, these are indispensable in modifying problem behaviors. However, the trainer you select should at least be fluent in the principles outlined in this book and have a thorough working knowledge of both fear-based and rank-based aggression problems and their resolution. This person should be able to speak with you intelligently about such topics as systematic desensitization, counterconditioning, and rank management and should be willing to explain these concepts to you so that you thoroughly understand them. After all, you're the person who's going to have to implement these programs.

At the same time, avoid trainers who assure you that they use only positive methods and don't believe in corrections. Their approach will be as one-dimensional as that of the yank-and-jerk trainer, though for different reasons. On the whole, try to avoid trainers who sound dogmatic about "only" doing this and "never" doing that. When you ask a good trainer the question "What is your training philosophy?" the best answer you could hope for is some version of "It depends." A good trainer will have a toolbox of strategies from which to choose and the breadth of experience to know which combination will best lend itself to the resolution of your particular issues.

Moreover, avoid trainers who promise you that they can fix all behavior problems if you just pay them enough money. A good trainer will understand not only his or her own limitations but also the limitations of the situation and will be frank with you about them. And finally, in relation to resolving the specific behavior issues discussed earlier, I would hesitate to send the dog away for training. A great many of these issues are directly related to the relationship you have with your dog, and so you should work on them in the context of your life as it is. The only time sending him away for training might make sense would be with the understanding that it's only a beginning, and that you're committed to continuing the work your trainer starts during your dog's period away.

Now, if you've found a trainer or behaviorist who appears competent, and he or she, after working with your dog for some time, suggests that you find a new home for your dog, I strongly recommend taking that advice. No matter how you feel about your dog, you cannot put your new child at risk, because in the end both the child and the dog will pay the price. Finding him a new home without a child now will ensure that everyone lives happily ever after.

Chapter Three

A Seamless Transition

The most critical element in making the integration of your new child into your home as seamless and easy as possible is to introduce, well ahead of time, as many of the changes that this integration will certainly entail. This way, your dog will not associate these changes with the arrival of the baby and so won't have a reason to take a dim view of the newcomer. If prepared for properly, the arrival of your baby will appear to be, from the perspective of the dog, a mere hiccup in his routine. In an ideal world the new elements of his routine would be introduced three to four months or more before the delivery date.

In order to prepare for the upcoming change in your household, begin by thinking about what your house rules are going to be once your child is on the scene, and start implementing those rules today. If you will no longer want your dog on the bed, get him off now (see page 13). If you won't want him on the furniture, same thing (see page 13). If you don't want him begging at the table, stop that behavior now (see page 29). If he's a counter surfer, deal with it today (see page 29). If he'll have to be isolated for periods of time during the day, begin introducing such isolation now (see page 60). If you've skipped over the Doggie Twelve-Step Program, you might glance at it to see whether your dog possesses any dicey behaviors that you hadn't previously thought of, and that you may want to curb. The long and the short of it is this: start today what you'll need to have done tomorrow, and tomorrow will less likely bring trouble.

Dogs, Children, and Toys

Among the issues you'll want to think about is how to deal with your dog's toys. If your dog is possessive about objects, see page 70. You may have noticed that a great many dog toys bear a striking similarity to children's toys. If you don't want your dog to appropriate every toy that comes into the house, help him differentiate now what's his from what's not his. There are several ways to accomplish this. First, avoid buying toys for your dog that are too much like kids' toys.

My favorite dog toys are easily identifiable as such — for example, tennis balls; hard rubber toys that allow you to put food in them, such as Kong Toys, Planet Dog toys, Buster Food Cubes or Balls; hollow bones with marrow holes that can be stuffed with food; cornstarch bones; bully sticks; and so on. There are dozens of interesting dog toys on the market and more coming out all the time. Visit your local pet shop and see what's new and different. Second, don't have a million dog toys lying around. Let your dog have access to only two or three that are easily identifiable. Even if you've found eight or ten toys that your dog really likes, rotate them so they're not always scattered about the house. The more of his things he's used to having scattered around, the higher the likelihood that he's going to assume that anything lying around on the floor is his.

CANINE RULES OF POSSESSION

What's mine is mine and what's yours is mine is a dog's general theory of ownership unless otherwise instructed. The following list of dog property laws, gleaned from the Internet, pretty well sums it up.[1]

- If I like it, it's mine.
- If it's in my mouth, it's mine.
- If I can take it from you, it's mine.
- If I had it a little while ago, it's mine.
- If it's mine, it must never appear to be yours in any way.
- If I'm chewing something up, all the pieces are mine.
- If it just looks like mine, it's mine.
- If I saw it first, it's mine.
- If you are playing with something and you put it down, it automatically becomes mine.
- If it's broken, it's yours.

Simplify your dog's life by (a) teaching him that everything is yours, and (b) getting him toys that he can easily distinguish from your child's toys and teaching him the difference between the two.

Finally, you can teach him to distinguish his toys from children's toys by taking advantage of his powerful sense of smell. To do this, begin practicing the following simple exercise. Start with two piles of toys — one a child's pile and one a dog's pile — separated by a few feet. On the toys in the child's pile, put a dab of Listerine so your dog can begin to build a scent association with these toys. Then, every time your dog approaches the child's pile, issue the command "off" (see page 29 if your dog doesn't know this command). If he approaches his own pile, praise him. Try this at different times of the day in different parts of the house with different groups of toys. Once he's good at this exercise, begin moving the two piles closer and closer together until they're right next to each other. Continue to use the "off" command if he even thinks about picking up a child's toy.

Once he's *really* good at this, it's time to increase the difficulty quotient. Mix together the toys in the two piles. Once again, if he shows interest in a child's toy he gets the command "off," and if he goes for one of his own toys he's a good boy. Continue to practice this exercise until you bring home your new baby. Each time you buy a new child's toy, put a dab of Listerine on it, show it to your dog while giving him the command "off," and then add it to your growing collection of toys. Your dog will soon figure out what's his and what isn't, and so long as you keep his own toy pile interesting, especially by stuffing some items with food, you shouldn't have any trouble.

The Child's Room and Other Zones

Something else to consider is the demarcation of certain zones in the house where your dog will have limited access. For instance, your new child's room, areas where you're planning to nurse your child, the space around his high chair, and finally, the space around the baby himself are all places in which the dog should be conditioned to follow certain rules. Let's go through this list and see what you can do to define these zones.

In my view, the child's room should be an area that your dog can access only with your permission. You want him to understand that this is not a playground, a resting area, or an area in any way available to him unless he has your okay. This will not only build in a necessary safeguard, but it will also allow you to teach him to form positive associations with this room and, by extension, with your child — but more on that in a moment.

THE ZONE DEFENSE

Teaching your dog to respect certain zones around your child will build a huge safety margin into their relationship. It will also give you great latitude in controlling your dog's interactions with your child and in using them to cultivate in your dog both propriety and a positive outlook on the whole situation.

Right now, let's talk about teaching him that he's never to enter this room without your permission. I'll run down a number of methods you can use. I suggest working with them all simply to ensure that your dog really gets it. Begin by having your dog on a leash with a training collar (see the appendix for a discussion of collars). Then walk him near the baby's future room and begin throwing treats on the floor *outside the room*, allowing your dog to get them. Throw six to eight treats down, so that your dog is really into it, and then suddenly toss the next one into the child's room. Most dogs will charge right toward the room; as he approaches the threshold, give him a quick nudge on the collar combined with a sharp "no." The level of force you use should be tempered to the sensitivity of your dog. You should find the level that's just strong enough to get the job done the first time around. Anything more is excessively harsh — as is anything less, since you'll merely have to give the correction more often.

Of course, when this happens the first time, your dog will be somewhat surprised and will try to figure out why he got corrected. To help him out, continue to throw treats on the floor *on your side of the door* and once again encourage him to get them. After he's had enough treats to get him excited once more, toss another one into the room and repeat the correction. As soon as your dog has been corrected, once again start throwing him treats on your side of the door. What you're doing is playing a game I call "identify the variable." You want him to figure out what the difference is between the treats on your side of the door and those on the other side — and of course, the door is the difference. It's important to bring your dog back to taking treats on your side of the door as soon as possible after his correction in order to both restore his positive mood and teach him that it's not the treats themselves that are the problem. It's crossing the threshold.

You'll be amazed at how fast most dogs pick this up. Usually three to five repetitions and the dog starts getting it. To fully develop this behavior, the first time you throw a treat into the room and your dog hesitates to go in, you should *immediately praise him wildly* and offer him a treat from your hand. You want to highlight for him the moment he got it right, not simply through the lack of a correction but through a highly positive consequence as well.

Once your dog gets this, you should make things a bit more complicated for him. If he has a favorite toy, like a tennis ball that he likes to chase, give him a few throws near the baby's room and then suddenly throw one right into the room. If he attempts to go in the room to retrieve the toy, he gets a correction; and if he refuses to enter he gets wildly praised and perhaps is even rewarded with a treat. Once your dog understands these exercises, try periodically walking him past the baby's room and suddenly, outside of what he can identify as a training situation and without warning, throw a treat or a favorite toy into the room. At this point, if he attempts to enter the room, a sharp verbal command should do the trick, so you should be able to do this without a leash. If you can't, then you should go back and redo the first stages of the exercise until a verbal reprimand is all you need. Ultimately you should need no reprimand whatsoever, since your dog will have learned never to go into that room.

When your dog has thoroughly understood this exercise, you can work the entire concept from a new angle. Of course, the more angles from which you work this, the more solidly your dog will understand what you're trying to teach him. With your dog on the outside of the room, put a few favorite family members or friends inside. Then have them do anything they can to entice the dog to come into the room, *aside from actually calling him to come.* They should make high-pitched squeaky sounds, toss his favorite toy around inside the room, look at him, tell him what a good boy he is, and generally

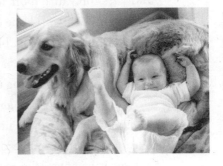

attempt to be as interesting to him as possible. You should be in the room also, and if your dog attempts to cross the threshold immediately verbally reprimand him and give him a quick squirt of water on the nose. Now, this may seem inherently unfair, but remember, you're trying to teach him that no matter what it looks like, he's simply not allowed in that room, period. Keep in mind that one day your child might be rolling around on the floor laughing and looking like a perfect playmate for your dog. Won't it be nice to know that your dog would never go in there unless you give him permission?

A final exercise that will really nail this behavior down involves the use of a ScatMat, a rubber mat with a harmless yet annoying static pulse running through it. Lay this mat down right in front of the door to the child's room and turn it on. This is ideal if your dog is the type who will attempt to go into the room as soon as you're not in the area. The moment he steps on the mat, he'll get a surprising static pulse on his feet and will quickly learn to avoid the area. You can also tempt the dog to cross into the area as in the exercises described earlier. A couple of steps onto the mat will convince him that this is a bad idea. Once your dog gets this, be sure to leave the mat outside the door for at least a few weeks. Soon your dog will stop thinking of that room as a place he can enter, and most of your training goals will have been accomplished.

There is, however, one more thing. The idea here is not that the dog should never enter the room; *it's that he should learn never to enter that room without your permission, and ultimately, that it's a special place with special rules.* When he has really understood the first part (at least a few weeks should have gone by during which he hasn't attempted to enter the room and he's passed all your tests), you can teach him the second part also. If you're using a ScatMat, simply turn it off, leave it in place, invite the dog into the room with a command such as "Come on in," and then encourage him to enter. He may hesitate in the beginning, but continue to encourage him, even gently with the leash and a few treats, if necessary, until he comes along. When he walks across the mat and nothing unpleasant happens, he'll begin to realize that it's safe to enter the room *so long as you're with him and have given him specific permission.* Even if you're not using the ScatMat, the same principle applies: he learns that once you've given the okay, and only then, nothing unpleasant happens if he enters the room. As you will see in another section, this will come in handy when you make the baby's room into a special place with which he has all sorts of positive associations.

Once your dog has learned to enter the baby's room only with your okay, you can add another element. After bringing him into the room, have him do obedience exercises for you there. Teach him to associate this context with taking direction from you. Never let him get the sense that this is a free-for-all play area. In particular, it's a good idea to have a special place, like a dog bed, in the room on which he's learned to spend a good bit of time in a down-stay. Teach him to associate this room with controlled behavior now, and once your child arrives such behavior will be second nature to him.

Now that we've defined the baby's room as a special zone, think about other areas where the same controlled behavior would be useful and begin to define those as special zones now. Areas where you think you'll be nursing your child fall into this category. So does the child's high chair. Defining certain areas as special zones is not particularly difficult, but as with everything else, a little diligence and persistence are required.

As in the case of boundary training in the child's room, setups are the key. Identify the zone you'd like to outline, and begin using your squirt bottle and the command "out" to enforce its boundaries. Every time your dog enters the area (generally within a five- to six-foot circle around the object) give the command "out" in a firm tone. If your dog does not immediately leave the area, he gets a quick squirt from either the water bottle or the now-hated Bitter Apple spray or Pet Corrector. A few repetitions of this should give him the idea, and he should be especially responsive if you've done all or most of the other things outlined in this book so far. He'll be so receptive to taking direction from you that, at this point, a little should go a long way.

SITUATIONAL LEARNING

As you may have already learned, situational learning can work both for you and against you. In this case, it will work for you as your dog begins to associate situations in which your child is present with acceptable and positive behaviors.

When your child is especially young, you'll want to define his nursing areas in this manner, but as he gets older his high chair will become his central feeding place. While, as we'll see shortly, it's all right to invite your dog to enter the zone and calmly lie next to you when you're nursing, I recommend that, once your child starts using a high chair, you never let your dog into the eating zone. That's because little children are notoriously messy eaters, and once they're in a high chair there will be food flying in all directions. This will only get worse as your child gets older. If your dog is in the eating zone he'll quickly learn that the child's eating area is a great place for table scraps.

"So what?" you might say to yourself. "If the dog eats the mess I won't have to clean it up." That might be true, but I'd prefer that your dog didn't view your child as a source of food. It won't take a huge stretch of your dog's imagination for him to continue to view your child in this way. Once Junior becomes more mobile and starts running around the house with cookies in hand, it'll be tempting for your dog to resort to highway robbery and steal things from him. If he learns to see this obviously helpless and uncoordinated little child as a lower-ranking pack member and a source of food, a competitive dynamic may be set in motion that can be the source of serious behavior problems. You can avoid all of this by simply teaching your dog to respect the child's eating zones exactly in the way he should respect yours.

That said, I do think that having your dog associate your child with food and treats in a controlled context can be helpful in developing a friendly and nurturing relationship between them. In the context of the high chair, this would simply mean that, on the one hand, while your child is eating, your dog is not permitted to raid food from the zone around the child's chair. And on the other, when your child is done eating, you can give your dog permission to clean up. In this manner you can encourage self-control and respect on the part of your dog at the same time that you use the food scraps to help him develop a positive view of your child, who has now become a source of goodies but not a pushover.

The Stroller

Soon a stroller is going to become a semipermanent feature of your life and that of your dog, so you might as well begin introducing it now. Not only do you want your dog to be familiar with the stroller visually, but you also want her to learn how to walk next to it without pulling or lunging. A dog who lunges and pulls on the leash while you're walking your child in a stroller is dangerous and will have to stay home. Of course, the foundation of proper leash behavior is the pay-attention game, described on page 21. Before you can even think about letting your dog accompany you when you take your child out in the stroller, your dog must master this exercise. Once she has, the rest is a piece of cake.

To prepare your dog to walk calmly next to the stroller, simply take her out with it as often as possible before the baby's due date. Since in this situation you won't be in a position to do the sudden turnarounds described in the training exercise in chapter 1, simple nudges on the leash will have to do. With your stroller empty, you won't have to worry about endangering your baby while working with your dog. As you walk along with your dog and stroller, teach your dog to maintain a position near you and behind the stroller's threshold. It doesn't matter which side you tell her to walk on, but consistently sticking to one side would be helpful. If your dog steps beyond the threshold, give a quick leash nudge accompanied by a verbal reprimand such as "no" or "uh-uh-uh."

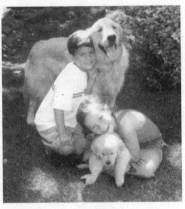

Photo: Belinda Levinson

Once she's learned to stay near you and is walking appropriately, teach her to associate that position with a word or phrase, such as "with me," as well as with an occasional treat. If your dog learns that good things happen to her within the zone you've designated as appropriate, she's likely to want to hang around in there. *When you feel that she understands this concept,* hold her responsible for obeying it; give her a leash nudge if she fails to comply after she's heard your "with me" command. What you'll find is that soon your dog will learn to associate the presence of the stroller with controlled walking, and you'll no longer need to use any verbal cues. Practice this diligently in the weeks or months before your child enters your life, and going for a walk will present no problems when there is finally a baby in the stroller.

A Little Theater

The following exercise requires a bit of theater. While seemingly silly it's one more way to prepare both you and your dog for the very real changes that are heading your way.

Begin by buying a doll that is about the size of an actual baby. This is going to be your surrogate child until the real thing arrives, and it will condition your dog to the sight of you carrying a bundle like this around. Additionally, it will enable you to teach him how to behave around this bundle. To make your performance more compelling, see if you can acquire a blanket that already has the scent of an infant on it. Often hospitals have used receiving blankets on hand, and the staff at your local hospital may be willing to part with one. Otherwise, if you have friends with a small child, perhaps you could give them a fresh blanket that they could use for a few days and then return to you fully scented. The idea, of course, is to swaddle the doll in this blanket and relate to it in front of your dog as if it were the genuine article.

Start carrying the faux baby around with you to get a sense of what you'll soon be dealing with. This will allow you to notice the places where you will most likely want to set your child down. Those are places that you should define as special zones, just as you defined the baby's room and areas where the baby will be nursed as special zones. Additionally, *the doll itself should have a permanent zone around it.* Teaching this to your dog is simple, especially if you've already done everything outlined earlier. Whenever you set the doll down, use your squirt bottle and the "out" command to teach your dog that he's not allowed near the doll without your permission. Of course, you should occasionally let him sniff the "baby" so that he can familiarize himself with the scent, and if you first command him to sit before you allow him a sniff, so much the better. The idea, of course, is to teach your dog respect and propriety in relation to both the bundle in your hand and its scent.

Another benefit of this exercise is that it will condition you and your dog to the changes in body posture that you will adopt when you have a baby to carry. Since dogs are acutely aware of body posture, it's important that your dog becomes used to the new shape that your body will take on as you use backpacks, slings, and carriers of various sorts (some dogs might spook with the sudden change and will need acclimation). It's also important that you communicate effectively with your dog even when burdened with your baby. Practice both sitting and walking around with the doll in your arms, in a sling, or in a BabyBjörn, and in any other situations or positions you can think of. Then pay attention to how this affects your ability to interact with your dog and how your dog relates to you while you're in these positions. For most dogs, none of this will make much difference, but for some it will. You should know which camp your dog falls into long before your baby's arrival.

Photo: Belinda Levinson

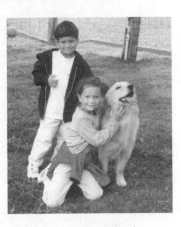

Finally — and this should be obvious — don't do what some recent clients of mine mistakenly did, which was to bring home a baby blanket and throw it on the floor for the dogs to use as a toy. Duh! But apparently such things need to be pointed out. These folks thought that letting their dogs pee on and then tear up the blanket would be a great way to familiarize them with the scent. When one of the dogs bit their child in the face, predictably at the age of eight months, the parents were surprised, but they shouldn't have been. Teach your dog the right associations from early on.

Other Baby Sights, Sounds, and Smells

While introducing the baby doll, it's a good idea to familiarize your dog with other items that will soon become common in your life, such as car seats, swings, and noisy baby toys, among others. As you bring home new items, introduce them one or two at a time and gauge your dog's reaction. If your dog appears spooked by something like a high chair or a swing suspended in a doorway, leave these items set up in the places where they are likely to remain, and allow your dog to become acclimated to them.

MOTORIZED BABY SWINGS

If you are considering using a motorized baby swing, a word of caution is in order. In a number of cases, dogs have pulled young children out of such swings and killed them. Apparently the sound of the swing triggered the dogs' prey instinct, and the parents, thinking their children were safe in their swings, were not nearby. If you are planning to use such a swing, install it as early as possible and acclimate your dog to it consistently, gauging his response all the way along. And of course, never leave your dog unsupervised with your child!

If your dog is extremely shy but food-motivated, then repeatedly lace the area surrounding the new item, and perhaps the item itself, with treats, until she becomes accustomed to it. This is especially important with toys that have flashing lights and make odd sounds (more on baby-related noises in a moment). Each time you turn them on, deliver yummy treats to your dog. Continue to do this until she develops a powerfully positive association with them. And when introducing scary new items, be sure to use an upbeat tone of voice with your dog to illustrate that there's nothing to fear. Using a soothing or coddling tone of voice, a common response when faced with a fearful dog, will usually make the problem worse. Never comfort, coddle, or reassure a fearful dog in any way! Again, adopt an upbeat and happy tone to help convince your dog that all is well.

If your dog is easily spooked by strange sounds, you might also consider buying one of the many CDs of recorded baby sounds that are available and play it often. The best way to introduce it is to play the CD at a low volume while you are doing something with your dog that she enjoys immensely — treats, games, or cuddling with you. Then, over time, slowly increase the volume until it's at the level of ordinary baby sounds. When desensitizing your dog to anything, it is always important to avoid crossing her fear threshold, if possible. If you notice her becoming agitated at the baby sounds, simply turn the volume down a bit and continue at that level until she has become accustomed to it. Additionally, if your dog is extremely sensitive you can isolate her for a period of time before and after you listen to the baby sounds together, so that the interaction becomes an exciting and fun-filled period between two stretches of relative boredom.

With respect to strange new scents in your house, you can easily acclimate your dog to these by applying things like baby lotions, powders, creams, and shampoos to yourself to help your dog associate them with something familiar and comforting.

Learning to Accept Baby Movements

We have already discussed desensitizing your dog to childlike handling (page 37) and controlling his sleeping and resting areas. Let me add a couple of details about those subjects in order to fill out the picture.

First, since most of us relate to our dogs from either a standing or a sitting position, the notion of crawling may come as a surprise to some dogs. It's a good idea, then, to introduce this type of movement early on. There's not much to it. Simply get on the floor and crawl toward your dog, making friendly, playful noises and offering him a few pats and scratches on the head, as well as some treats if he seems uneasy. You can employ multiple members of your household in this. If your dog, rather than being taken aback by this, perceives it as a cue to become wild and playful to the degree that he gets physical with you, be sure to discourage this. Pop up quickly, issue a mild reprimand and ask him to comply with a few obedience commands in order to switch him to a more receptive and stable state of mind. Remember, you don't want your dog to view your baby as a crawling squeaky toy. If your baby has already arrived but is not yet in the crawling stage, try this approach: once you have done a little

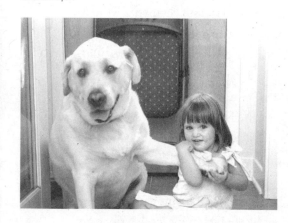

Photo: Bari Halperin

preliminary work to get your dog used to your crawling, place your child on your back with the help of a third party and do the same exercises. It won't take long for your dog to get the idea.

If your dog nonetheless finds the whole business alarming or (later, when the baby is crawling on his own) is simply not always in the mood to be crawled upon and handled by a baby, it is a good idea to teach him that he can leave the area and retreat to a safe place. Of course, in order to do that you need to help define a safe place for your dog — a place to which he can retreat and to which your child won't have access. This could be a crate, an area of the house cordoned off with baby gates, the backyard, or anything else you can think of. If you have done ample desensitizing exercises to teach your dog to accept childlike handling, but your dog still gets nervous or a bit tired of your child's approaches, teach him a phrase such as "take a break" to let him know he can retreat to a safe place as an indication that he's had enough.

Accomplishing this is reasonably straightforward. Before your baby's arrival, when you've had a chance to play with your dog and you sense that he's getting tired, say to him, "Take a break," and, with a treat, guide him to a designated safe area. Give him his treat and then a nice bone or other high-value object that will keep him busy for a while and help him settle down in this special area. After your baby has arrived, employ this same routine when you sense your dog has had enough. In this way you'll teach him that he has the option to retreat, that he doesn't have to suffer through handling at times when he finds it irritating.

The Dog Who Is Always Underfoot

Some dogs are so clingy that they seem to always be underfoot. Of course, with a baby in your arms or a toddler stumbling along next to you, this can get annoying. So it makes sense to teach your dog to give you some personal space when you demand it.

Doing so is relatively simple. Choose a cue such as the word *out* and issue it when your dog is underfoot. Then enforce it with a twofold, carrot-and-stick approach. With your dog underfoot say, "Out," in a commanding tone, and then toss a few treats out about ten feet away from you. Naturally your dog will run out to grab the treats. Once she's eaten the treats, though, she's likely to want to return to the underfoot position. As she approaches, give her the command "out" again, and if she continues to approach give her a quick squirt with a water bottle, some Bitter Apple spray, or a blast from the Pet Corrector, as described in previous sections. When she retreats again, toss a few more treats beyond the designated "out" zone to reward her for staying there.

Soon you will see that she hesitates to approach. Once she has learned to keep her distance, continue to toss treats beyond the "out" zone. In time, reduce the treats and then eliminate them altogether, since in the end you want your dog simply to get out of the zone upon request, without the use of gimmicks. If you practice this frequently, long before the arrival of your child, your dog will be unlikely to associate the "out" command with your child's presence.

As the Big Day Gets Closer

As the baby's due date approaches, if you have dealt with potential problem behaviors and have had a chance to implement a good deal of what's been discussed so far, then you're in the home stretch. Everything should be dovetailing nicely.

Let's talk about some things you can do during the last month or so to be sure that you're totally prepared on the day your baby comes home. If you haven't already done so — or not as much as you would have liked — begin tapering off the amount of attention you're giving your dog. Bring this to a level commensurate with the amount you're going to be able to give him once the baby arrives. Definitely avoid the temptation to indulge your dog in one last hurrah, knowing that soon you won't have the kind of time for him that you've had in the past. *Overindulging him now is the single quickest way to cause your dog to have an emotional meltdown once your child arrives, and in some cases the damage can be irreversible.* (Irreversible usually means the dog gets a new home or is euthanized.)

If you find that in the context of tapering the level of attention you give your dog, he is not getting the exercise he needs, now might be the time to consider enlisting the services of a dog walker.

A LITTLE HELP, PLEASE!

Dog walkers and other pet professionals are definitely people whose services you should consider enlisting. Their help can take an enormous amount of pressure off you and, in many instances, will make the difference between a smooth transition and a disaster. Find a reputable person by asking around at your vet's and talking to people at the local dog park. Satisfied customers are happy to share their experiences, and you want to find someone with lots of satisfied customers.

A good dog walker will take your dog out daily with a group of other dogs to a safe, off-leash play area for an hour or so. There they will romp around, chase balls, wrestle, and so on, and when your dog comes home he should be thoroughly exhausted. This will take the pressure off you, as the dog's primary source of entertainment. Doing this at least a month before your child arrives will ensure that your dog is comfortable with both his walker and the dogs in his play group when the big day comes.

In conjunction with this, it would also be a good idea to get your dog used to spending some time alone in the house in an isolated area, such as in a crate, behind a baby gate in the kitchen, in the backyard, or in some other area where he does not have access to you. I can guarantee that there are going to be times when you simply want him out of your hair. A few daily periods of isolation should become a part of your dog's routine. (If your dog has issues with separation anxiety, see page 60.) Of course, a special bone for him during these periods wouldn't hurt. And finally, it wouldn't be a bad idea to teach your dog to occasionally stay in a kennel or with a friend. If you haven't done so already, now would be a good time to introduce this as well. This will be particularly helpful on the day your child arrives, as you will see in a moment.

As difficult as it may be, imagine what your life is going to look like once you have a child; then, condition your dog to that set of circumstances as soon as possible. If you do this, the arrival of the baby will seem like a mere bump in the road in your dog's routine, and he won't have the opportunity to develop negative associations with the addition of his new pack member. Begin this work as far ahead of your baby's due date as possible; that way, there will be less for you to think about regarding your dog once your child is here. This is a good thing, because, frankly, once your child is here you're going to have precious few moments to think of anything other than him or her. Let's take a look at how to handle the big day and the months after.

The Moment of Truth

With all the preparations made, you and your dog are now ready for the big event. As the baby's due date becomes imminent, you'll want to start thinking about what you're going to do with your dog while you're giving birth. I recommend that you take advantage of the fact that he's been conditioned to periodically boarding at a kennel or staying with a friend and put him there during this critical period. Even if your birth takes place at home, I still recommend this. The birth process is notoriously unpredictable, and knowing that your dog is in the good hands of someone else can add at least a little to your peace of mind during this time. That way, your focus will be on the arrival of your child, and not what's going on with your dog.

If you aren't in a position to do this, then be sure that your dog walker takes the dog out for extra long outings on the days surrounding the delivery, keeping him both busy and exhausted. This way, even if you're gone for an unusually long time your dog will probably sleep right through it. If the dog-walker option is also not a possibility for you, then hopefully you will have conditioned your dog to occasionally tolerate long periods of time home alone. Whatever the case, you should now be in a position not to have to give your dog a second thought while your child is making his or her debut in this world.

With the debut made, the time for the introduction is at hand. If, as you come home, your dog is there awaiting your arrival, begin by letting any friends or family members accompanying you enter the house first so that your dog can express to them his full enthusiasm for your return and be appreciably settled down by the time he meets your child for the first time. If possible, when it's time for the introduction, have your dog leashed and handled by a friend or a member of the family. In the end this may not be necessary, but it never hurts to take precautions.

Photo: Mike Wombacher

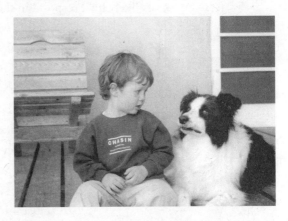

At this time, be calm, even nonchalant, about it. Ask your dog to sit, and then gently bring your baby down and let him to have a sniff and a look, starting at the feet. After a few moments of sniffing, tell him he's a good dog and then go about your business. Don't make a big deal of it. Treat the whole thing calmly. Later, when you have settled in a bit you can extend the introduction. Sit down on the sofa and let your dog sniff your baby's feet again, then ask for compliance with a command before allowing him to do a little more sniffing. And so on. At length, ask your dog to lie down nearby, give him a yummy chewy of some sort, and continue to hang out with him. Throughout all this, be sure not to express any nervousness or anxiety, because this can easily be transmitted to your dog. Express calm joy, and your dog will likely experience that as well. If you have done the exercises outlined so far, this introduction should present no significant problems.

For example, if you have done the exercises with your dog and the baby doll (see page 106), your dog will have learned to gently sniff the little bundle with no jumping or pushy licking behaviors. Of course, he is not stupid. He will immediately recognize that there is a universe of difference between the inanimate doll and the very much alive child in your arms. But his previous experience in the earlier situation will supply a "template" for his behavior now, and most likely he'll respond in the manner that you've taught him.

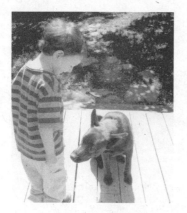

Photo: Jane Reed

Similarly, when you put your child in his room or crib, your dog should have learned his boundaries and should naturally keep a respectful distance. If you'd like, you might invite him into the area, but it should always be in a controlled manner. Since you've taught him to associate these areas with obedience commands previously, he will expect to have to perform them now. Be sure to meet his expectations. Keep him in a sit-stay or a down-stay, and don't forget to praise him when he complies. It's easy to ignore good behavior and miss precious opportunities to positively reinforce the dog for behaviors you like.

Once your child has been home a little while, the introductions have been made, and you're somewhat settled in, it might be a good time to put your dog in his special area so that he's simply out of the way. This, too, is something that he will have learned to expect and should have no trouble complying with. In fact, all that you ask of your dog now should be so thoroughly in line with what he has learned previously that, as I've said, he'll view the baby's arrival as not that big a deal.

Once the first day is behind you, you should simply continue with the routine you've established. Since your dog has learned to expect less of your attention, he won't feel suddenly ostracized now. He'll expect to see his dog walker at midday. He'll be used to spending a part of the day alone in a special area. And he will have learned appropriate behaviors in relation to special zones in the house.

The next step is to teach him to build positive associations with the presence of your child. In order to do this, try something that may initially seem counterintuitive: spend as much time as you can with your dog in the presence of your child and significantly less time with him in the absence of your child.

Many people are inclined to instead spend some time playing with their dog once their child is sleeping or otherwise occupied, and to put their dog in another room when they tend to their child's needs. Of course, to some degree there's no problem with that. But quiet moments of attention to and affection with your child should routinely take place with your dog involved. Since you've been toning down your interactions with your dog in preparation for your child's arrival, your attention will now have become, from the dog's perspective, an especially valued resource. When you give your dog access to your attention primarily in the presence of your child, he will naturally view your child's presence as something positive. Additionally, since you've taught him appropriate behaviors in relation to your child's presence, these will be positively reinforced and continually strengthened by the affection he receives in this context. Let's take a look at all this in practical terms.

Say you're going to your child's room to play with him or to do something functional like change his diapers. Invite your dog to join you. Recall that you have previously taught him to associate that room with obedience commands and docile behavior. Once he's in, give your dog some attention in the form of a few quick obedience commands, reward him with a little affection, and ask him to lie down on the dog bed, to which you have already accustomed him, and stay there. Attend to your child, but periodically take a few moments to verbally and, if possible, physically praise your dog. An occasional treat wouldn't hurt either. Go back and forth between your child and the dog as seems appropriate. Of course, if before you brought the dog into this interaction he was alone for some period of time, he will undoubtedly view it in a positive light. And that is the whole point — to teach your dog to develop deep, powerfully positive associations with your child's presence.

Another effective way to build positive associations with the presence of your child involves the use of a carrier or sling, such as the BabyBjörn type. With your child strapped to your chest, interact with your dog in the form of petting and stroking interspersed with some light obedience exercises. Here, too, if your dog has been relatively alone before this interaction, he will naturally view this playful "family time" in an extremely positive light: the presence of your child means fun and affection for him.

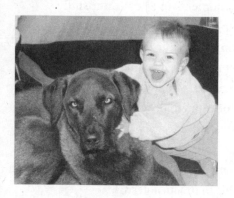

Photo: Mike Wombacher

Of course, such exercises have the added benefit of teaching your dog to associate the presence of your child with your authority and control. With that in mind, be sure to work in the handling exercises described on page 37. And if you perform the exercises around the food dish and other objects he considers his own (see page 72), this effect will be even further enhanced. The more you can do to teach your dog to associate your child both with affectionate and playful interactions and with your authority, the better prepared you will be for the eight-month threshold — when your child will become mobile, first by crawling, then by walking. As mentioned earlier, this is usually when, in the absence of appropriate preparatory steps, real problems between dogs and children tend to emerge.

The point is, too many people teach their dogs that, when the baby is around, they're in the proverbial doghouse: the presence of the child comes to mean the absence of attention for the dog. Having prepared in the way I've described allows you to reverse this situation and teach your dog that the presence of your child means affection and structured play for him. Any time that you spend with your child is an opportunity to deepen the bond between your child, your dog, and yourself.

When the time comes to wind down the interaction with your child, it's a good idea to make a point of returning your dog to his special place as well, give him something yummy to chew on, and go about your business. Again, this drives home the point that your child's presence means your presence and lots of fun interactions, and that your child's absence often means quiet time for him — a powerful way to build deeply positive associations.

There is one final rule that should be obeyed without exception: *No unsupervised interactions between your dog and your child — ever! Period.* This is an absolute rule and should remain in effect for years. It takes only a second for something to go wrong, and that second could change your life forever. Despite all the good training you've done, you should never take anything for granted, because mistakes happen. Your dog could inadvertently knock your child over, or he could grab for a toy at the same time your child does so and may accidentally bite your child's hand. If you're not there, you'll never know exactly what happened. Who will pay the price? Your dog, of course, since you will no longer trust him, a fact that may throw your whole relationship up in the air. If you are not in a position to supervise the interactions between your dog and your child, then separate them. That way you can be assured that nothing unfortunate will happen.

The Importance of Supervision

Years ago, a newspaper article told the following story. A mother was working in the kitchen, about six feet away from her two-year-old daughter and six-year-old

Rottweiler. She took her eyes off the two playmates for two seconds, and during those two seconds the child spilled a bag of potato chips on the floor and then tried to pick them up. Since they'd fallen right at the dog's feet, a confrontation developed and the dog severely bit the child, causing life-threatening injuries that would require many years and numerous surgeries to repair.

This dog had previously never shown a propensity for violence and was by all accounts a nice dog. Unfortunately the mother had made two mistakes: she had never taught the dog not to consider objects his own, and she had taken her eyes off the child and dog, even if only for two seconds. Never forget that it takes only two seconds for something to go horribly wrong.

Another story, one that happened in London years ago, highlights a different aspect of the issue of supervision. A mother had left her three-year-old son in his bedroom with the family Labrador, by all accounts an amiable fellow who had never shown the slightest sign of trouble with the child. As the mother was working in the kitchen, she heard a cry from the bedroom. When she rushed in, she noticed that her son had several puncture wounds in his face. Horrified, she had her dog euthanized the next day and asked the vet to perform an autopsy to help determine why her dog had gone crazy.

During the autopsy the vet pulled crayons out of both of the dog's ears. What a tragedy! When it comes to dogs and young children, neither party is trustworthy and both may end up paying a price. Always supervise the interactions between your dog and your small child, no matter how safe leaving them alone together may seem.

After the Eight-Month Threshold, and Looking into the Future

As I've suggested, the true test of whether all your work has been successful is the day your child becomes mobile, which will most likely happen when he reaches around eight months of age. At that point the interactions between your dog and your child will become more frequent and unpredictable. Even with the best supervision, the unexpected is guaranteed. If you have diligently followed the recommendations I've discussed so far, there likely won't be any problems. But never be too bold in your assumptions. Don't make the mistake of letting down your guard.

As your child grows, the exercises you do with him and your dog should evolve. Continue to regularly do the handling exercises discussed on page 118, with your child in a BabyBjörn or, if he's getting too big for that, in your lap. Once he's old enough — perhaps around two or three years of age — have him begin to give simple obedience commands to your dog with you there to enforce them. You can start by standing behind your child like a puppeteer and actually forming the hand signals with his hands while both of you issue simple commands, such as "sit." If your dog refuses to comply, gently but firmly demand compliance. If he does comply, have your child give him a treat (if he is capable of doing so — if not, then you supply the reward). Continue to do this until your child is old enough to stand on his own in front of your dog and issue the commands.

At that point, you should minimize your dog's awareness of yourself and increasingly focus his attention on your child. The best way to accomplish this is to begin by leashing your dog and standing by his side as your child gives simple commands. Again, if your dog complies, either

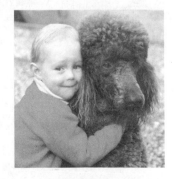

Photo: Kimberly Burke

you or (preferably) your child should reward him with both a treat and affection. Once your dog is routinely responding to the child's commands, begin taking up a position behind the dog instead of standing beside him. This will place your dog's focus entirely on your child, who should continue to give the command and hand signal to the best of his ability. And if your dog complies, he receives a yummy treat from your child. If he does not, you will gently but quickly enforce the command.

Of course, by the time you've gotten to the point where you're able to stand behind your dog and have your child give him direction, your dog will have had so many exposures to this that he should have it down pat. Continuing to do these exercises over the years, as your child gets older, is the best way to ensure both that your child learns appropriate ways of relating to your dog and that your dog learns to respond with respect.

It should be clear that in conjunction with such exercises your child should be taught kindness and self-control. It's unreasonable to expect your dog — no matter how gentle a soul he may be — to tolerate endless harassment from a young child who is incapable of appreciating the consequences

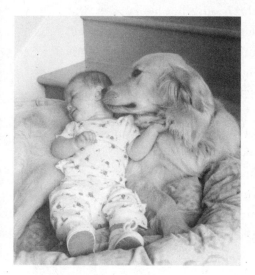

of his actions. This is an important part of your child's education and will help him enormously when he encounters dogs other than yours. To put it bluntly, no matter how tolerant your dog is, you must teach your child not to kick, pull, pinch, poke, or otherwise tease or torment him. This should be obvious. Nonetheless, you'll have to be diligent here, since most children are notoriously resistant to being scolded for such activity — which is why I recommend that you never leave a child with a dog unsupervised. Also bear in mind that even if your dog has the tolerance of a Buddhist monk when subjected to your child's teasing, *another dog may not.* And this can lead to dangerous consequences for a child who cannot appreciate the difference.

Along the same lines, teach your child never to suddenly jump on or surprise the dog while he's dead asleep or otherwise unaware of the child's presence. There's no telling how even the most well-behaved dog will respond when startled and scared.

In short, teach your child to always pet your dog in ways that are pleasurable and acceptable to him and to avoid inadvertently or intentionally tormenting him. Of course, if you've conditioned your dog to tolerate all kinds of rough handling, using the exercises described on page 37, and you've taught your child how to handle your dog appropriately, you've worked the problem from both ends — and this should lead to a safe and appropriate relationship between the two of them.

In a perfect world your child will not merely be petting your dog or practicing simple obedience exercises. The two of them will also be playing games. There are a few rules to bear in mind here. First, avoid having your child play strength or competitive games with your dog, such as tug-of-war and chase. While they're okay for an adult who can initiate, control, and end such games (as described on page 36), it won't take long for your dog to figure out that he's quicker and stronger than your child. This is information he can definitely live without. The last thing you want to do is to foster a physically confrontational and competitive atmosphere in your interspecies pack. Rather, you want to cultivate a relationship based on mutual respect and self-control. With that in mind, the best games for your child to play with your dog entail fetching, obedience exercises, and tricks.

Tricks in particular are a great way to have your dog and your child interact. Most kids are thrilled to see their dog doing tricks, and most dogs like doing them. They should be a source of lighthearted fun and entertainment for all concerned. So feel free to teach as many as you can manage.[2]

Hide-and-Seek

An excellent obedience game that involves calling the dog is hide-and-seek. You can begin this early on with two adults and one child. Begin by having the adults — one with the baby nearby — stand perhaps thirty feet apart. Then have the adult with the child call the dog. As soon as the command is issued, the adult holding the dog says, in a happy tone, "Go to…" — let's call her Caitlin — and the dog is released. As soon as she arrives at the adult with Caitlin, the dog receives a yummy treat from Caitlin's hand (probably held in the adult's hand). Then the dog is recalled to the first adult, where she receives another treat. The process is repeated several times, but each time the distance between the first adult and the adult with Caitlin increases. The first adult says, "Come," the second adult with the dog says, "Go to Caitlin," and the dog is released to be met by Caitlin and a treat on the other end.

Once this is well in hand, it is time to make two changes. The first is to drop the "Come" that has been issued by the adult with Caitlin. Now all the dog hears is "Go to Caitlin," upon which she is released. Having run through the exercise a number of times, the dog will fully understand what she is to do — go to Caitlin. And when she does she gets a treat. We have switched from a recall command to a "go to Caitlin" command. Once that is established, it's time to move even farther apart and to actually hide in an out-of-view room or closet. When the dog hears "Go to Caitlin," she has to find her before she gets her reward. So now you have a dog who is actively searching for Caitlin. And of course, when she finds her she gets a huge reward.

With respect to rewards, don't focus only on treats. If you have a dog who is ball or toy crazy, reward her with one of those. You (not your child, as noted earlier) can even reward her with a brief but intense game of tug-of-war (this is how search-and-rescue dogs are trained). If there are multiple members in your household, you can practice hide-and-seek with all of them, letting each in turn hide from the dog. If you persist, you will soon be able to tell your dog not only to "Go to Caitlin" but also to "Go to Johnny" or anyone else. As your Caitlin gets older, she will not need an adult to accompany her in this exercise. She'll be able to do it all on her own.

The recall exercise transformed into hide-and-seek is not only fun for your family but can also be a lifesaver if you ever find yourself in a real-life situation where you cannot locate your child. If your dog has learned to "go to Caitlin" in a fun environment at your house, she will also be able to do it at the park or anywhere else.

Other Issues

Before closing I'd like to cover a few additional areas that do not easily fall into the categories utilized above, but which are important enough to warrant your attention. They are organized in no particular order.

Two-Dog Households

If you have two dogs in your household, then the information in this book is, well, doubly pertinent. You will have to take stock of both of your dogs with respect to everything mentioned in these pages. Apply it as needed to bring them both into alignment with this program and, ideally, to make them equally obedient and generally responsive. In other words, everyone should be on the same page.

With two dogs, though, there are many more moving parts, and everything gets more chaotic. Of particular concern is how they play together. If your dogs like to roughhouse indoors — where they might knock over a stumbling toddler — be sure to begin teaching them to take it outside. Also, once your child arrives, keep an eye on the dogs' relationship with one another. Often a change in pack structure can trigger a competitive dynamic between two dogs, a dynamic that can have unpleasant consequences both for the dogs' relationship with each other and for their relationship with a child in the family. If you see such changes beginning to take place in your household, it is extremely important that you diligently implement the Doggie

Twelve-Step Program with both dogs, and that you have their complete re-spect. If you do have it, then as the pack leader you have the right to control interactions and conflict within your group. If you don't have it, the dogs may decide to settle their own issues, potentially with undesirable consequences.

Other People's Dogs

This brings us to another point. If you've done everything right, your child and your dog will develop an extraordinary relationship with one another, the memory of which will be with your child forever. However, there is one final area of concern worth considering. If your child lives with a friendly, easygoing dog at home, he is naturally going to assume that every dog he encounters out in the world is equally as easygoing — an assumption that can lead to disaster. Unfortunately there are dogs out and about who have no business mingling with the public. Should your child encounter one of them and presume that he's as friendly as your dog at home, things can get ugly fast. It's extremely important to teach him early how to relate to dogs he doesn't know.

Here are a few rules everyone should learn. First, teach your child never to approach a dog without being accompanied by an adult. Second, teach him that he should never approach any dog without asking you first. Dogs who are tied out in front of stores waiting for their owners should be avoided. You know nothing about them and don't want to make any casual assumptions simply because the dog seems friendly. If the dog is accompanied by an adult, be sure to ask whether he is friendly with children. *Never* let your child simply go up and pet the dog. If you sense *any* hesitation on the part of the adult, definitely pass. I continue to be amazed at the number of adults who simply ignore the hesitations or even outright warnings of dog owners and let their children approach the dog anyway. Such cavalier behavior can lead to disaster.

If the adult does give the okay, then have your child approach; but please observe a few basic rules about greeting strange dogs. Rather than letting your child approach the dog face to face, have him approach by offering his side to the dog and holding out a closed hand for him to sniff. Do not allow him to approach the dog suddenly or make abrupt movements. Teach him to approach part of the way and let the dog make up the difference by coming toward him. If the dog does not seem interested or show overt signs of friendliness, please pass on the encounter.

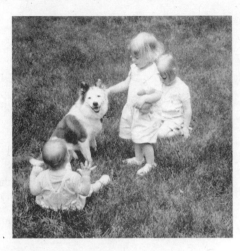

Photo: Katie Bracco

On the other hand, if he appears friendly and interested and approaches your child, have your child begin by petting him under the chin, not on the head, neck, or back. The latter areas are considered "socially sensitive" and may cause some dogs to take offense. A few gentle strokes under the chin are much more acceptable and much less risky. Also, direct face-to-face eye contact and hugs should be avoided at all costs, at least until a warm relationship is established between the two.

Finally, teach your child that if he sees a dog approaching, he should never run about and shriek or strike at the dog, as children are prone to do. Such behaviors may put the dog in either a play or a prey mode, either of which can result in injuries to your child. If a dog approaches, whether slowly or fast and whether friendly or not, your child should stand still even if he's scared. If he thinks for some reason that the dog might bite him, your child should put his clenched fists over his ears with his elbows coming down to his chest *and stand still!* The chances of any ill fortune befalling him under these circumstances are slim. Running around screaming and yelling will dramatically increase the likelihood of something unpleasant occurring, as will striking out at the dog.

RULES OF ENGAGEMENT

- Tell your child never to approach a dog without being accompanied by an adult.
- Your child should never approach a dog without asking you first.
- Always ask the adult who is accompanying the dog whether the dog is friendly. If the adult seems uncomfortable, please avoid interaction with the dog.
- If the adult gives the okay, have your child approach but also observe a few rules:
  - Ask your child to avoid face-to-face greetings.
  - Let him approach partway and then allow the dog to make up the difference.
  - If the dog does not appear to be interested, don't let your child continue to approach him.
  - Have your child pet the dog under the chin, not on the head, neck, or back; and please, no hugs.
- Teach your child not to run about wildly in the presence of a dog. If he becomes afraid of a dog, he should stand completely still and wait for the dog to lose interest or for someone to come and get him.

Following these simple guidelines will help ensure that your child's interactions with other people's dogs will always take place in a safe context and on a positive note.

Health and Hygiene

With all the things to think about while preparing for a baby's arrival, one that is often overlooked is the fact that in some ways a dog's health and a baby's health may be directly related. This is particularly true with respect to internal parasites such as worms, which are directly transmissible to children, as well as with respect to fleas, ticks, and mites, which are even more readily transmissible. It is also true of some skin conditions. It makes sense to take your dog for a thorough veterinary exam before your baby's arrival and to get routine health checks about once a year. You should also be sure to stock relevant preventive products such as antiflea medication if your situation requires it.

The need to keep your yard and other areas of your home free of dog poop should be self-evident. Be aware that dog excrement is loaded with germs that can cause all manner of health problems, including gastroenteritis. Similarly, be sure that bedding and carpeting is cleaned regularly so that what your dog drags inside is removed.

Additionally, it's always a good idea to make sure that your dog's nails are trimmed in order to prevent inadvertent scratches on your child, and, in the case of a shaggy dog, that his coat is regularly groomed and detangled. It is much easier for a young child to get her hands caught in a tangled coat and inadvertently pull the dog's hair, causing him annoyance and discomfort.

Geriatric Dogs and Dogs with Injuries

If you have a dog who is old and consequently in pain or suffering from dementia, or complete or partial blindness or deafness, you will have to take special precautions, especially once your child begins crawling. In such cases it is of the utmost importance to have a safe zone for your dog in order to protect both him and your child. Even the most amiable dog, when confused, sensorially deprived, or in pain, is likely to respond to inappropriate handling with displays of aggression, even if he has never exhibited aggression previously.

In the event that keeping the child and dog separated when not under close supervision becomes impossible, you should consider finding a new home for your dog. Bear in mind that as your dog's faculties gradually di-

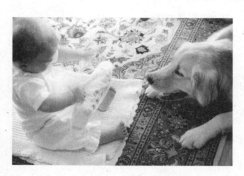

minish, your child's wildness will increase in tandem. As difficult as such a decision is, it is a lot less difficult than having to decide to euthanize your dog because he presents a danger to your child. If, when you find out that you are pregnant, you suspect that this might become an issue, then I recommend that you at least explore the new-home option with as many friends and family members as possible. Giving away an older dog is an emotionally trying and time-consuming process and, if required, one that you should embark on sooner rather than later.

A Few Final Thoughts

In these pages I've covered many ideas. On the one hand, making use of them may entail a lot of work, depending on your dog's behavior and disposition, but on the other hand it promises a wholesome and fulfilling relationship between your child and your dog. The payoff will continue for years and will make the work you have to put in on the front end more than worth it. I encourage you to make the effort to get it right.

If you find that you've followed the instructions in this book diligently but are still having problems with your dog in relation to your child, there are two possibilities. First, your dog may need more work with the lessons than you realized, and you should consider revisiting them. Second, it may be that your dog will never be entirely reliable with your child. In the latter case, I suggest finding the dog a new home as soon as possible. No matter how well in control you may believe you are, it's almost guaranteed that *if your dog is unreliable with your child, sooner or later something unpleasant will happen.* It's really just a matter of time. Such an event would result in both the child and the dog paying the price. By finding the dog a more appropriate home now, you'll do everyone a huge favor. Of course, before resorting to such a dramatic measure you should seek the advice of several professionals.

WHAT IF MY DOG EXHIBITS AGGRESSION TOWARD MY CHILD?

If your dog threatens your child, you should seek professional help for the dog *immediately*. There are also a couple of things to be aware of. First, never correct a dog for growling, showing his teeth, or displaying other warning signs. Issuing such a correction is likely to have unfortunate consequences: It will further impress upon your dog that the child's presence is undesirable, since now he has not only the experience of his own anxiety about your child's presence to deal with but also your anger. The presence of your baby is now doubly bad. Second, bear in mind that growling is a courtesy, a warning, and if you reprimand your dog for this courtesy he might dispense with it altogether, learning to bite without warning. Your dog will have no way to let you or anyone else know that he is anxious and feeling trapped, and he may decide to take the next step on his own.

I wish you the best of luck with the exciting events that are unfolding in your life. Few things provide a living connection to the mystery of what it means to be alive like the opportunity to be the vehicle by which a new life enters this world. The struggles that are involved in nurturing this new being and orienting her to her existence in this world pale by comparison to the joy of watching that little being as her potential unfolds. The fact that we participate in this mystery is extraordinary and the source of the deepest joy. Providing a wonderful home for a dog, that most loyal and devoted of animal companions, should only enrich this experience. With this in mind I leave you with best wishes and heartfelt blessings.

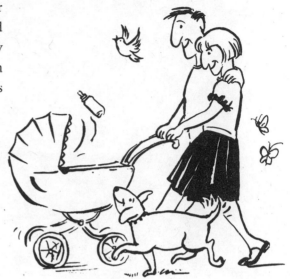

Appendix

Notes on Training Equipment

These days the question of training equipment has become laden with controversy. Let me share a few thoughts on the subject that may help you choose the appropriate equipment for your dog.

Years ago, when I first began training dogs, equipment was limited to various forms of choke chains, pinch collars (also known as prong collars), and a few different forms of harnesses. Since then a fair amount of new training equipment has entered the marketplace, including various forms of head collars and chest-led harnesses. What works for different dogs varies greatly, so you may have to experiment to see what is most suitable for your dog.

A few observations about each of these pieces of training equipment may help you get started. Choke chains are one type of equipment that I almost never use. Be aware that they are difficult to use properly and easy to use improperly. When used improperly they tend to create a band of steel around your dog's neck that compresses the soft tissue: the muscles, arteries, and trachea. And because, from the dog's perspective, the sensation is generally not that aversive, the chain may require a fair amount of force to achieve a desired response. Most often, a novice dog owner using a choke chain finds his dog dragging him down the street, the dog hacking and gagging as the chain compresses his neck.

Harnesses are safe, especially for small, delicate dogs, but they also tend to encourage pulling, which is precisely what, in a training context, we are trying to eliminate. The exception is the type of harness that has the leash clip at the front of the chest. If you are going to use a harness, I highly recommend this type. An ordinary harness with the leash clip at the dog's back is fastened around the strongest part of the dog's body; the dog will find it quite comfortable to pull against the leash with abandon. And dogs like to pull. That's why they put sled dogs in harnesses! A harness with the leash clip in front pulls the dog awkwardly off to one side when he pulls, in a way that dogs don't like. Consequently they tend to pull much less intensely or even stop pulling altogether.

Head collars fit around the dog's head like a bridle fits a horse. The purpose is to steer the dog's head gently and to simultaneously reduce or eliminate pulling. If the dog attempts to pull, this will cause his head to turn to one side or the other, and dogs don't like that. For some dogs, such a device works wonderfully. However, I have several issues with head collars and, except in rare cases, generally don't use them.[1] First, the head collar is not designed to allow you to give your dog a physical correction, and so it's primarily used by trainers who advocate a positive-only training methodology, in which any form of reprimand is considered tantamount to abuse. (As I mentioned earlier, I disagree with the basic premise of this approach.) But if you make the mistake of snapping the lead of a dog wearing a head collar, the chance that you will injure him is significant, because the snap will strongly torque his head to one side or the other. The same is true for the dog who continues to pull, albeit with less intensity, when wearing a head collar. The continued, long-term torque on the dog's neck can have negative health consequences in time.

What about pinch collars? In the last twenty years these collars have gotten an enormous amount of bad press for two reasons. First, they look like twelfth-century torture devices. And second, the politics of positive-only training have produced an avalanche of misinformation about them. The interesting thing about pinch collars is that, owing to their appearance, all their humane advantages are initially counterintuitive.

Let's take a look at what they don't do. They don't put a band of steel around your dog's neck that compresses the soft tissue. Rather, they pinch a little with rounded contact points, creating a superficial, nonchoking sensation that accomplishes two things. First, your dog has an organic reference point for that sensation because it mimics one way that dogs reprimand one another — by a quick bite on the neck. The collar takes advantage of a built-in set of responses in the dog that will make him pay attention quickly and does so in a way none of the other training gear mentioned here generally will. And second, because the sensation is immediately a little aversive, it takes only a fraction of the force required by any of the other pieces of equipment mentioned so far. To gain your dog's cooperation, pinch collars operate on about 5 percent of the level of force required by any other tool that's out there.

That said, any approach to training should not rely merely on the mechanics of training equipment. And no piece of training equipment is right for every dog. Feel free to experiment until you hit that right combination of equipment that works for you and your dog. And bear in mind that no training equipment is a substitute for a solid relationship built on the principles of mutual trust and respect.

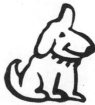

Notes

Introduction

1. "Dog Bites," Centers for Disease Control and Prevention, last updated September 5, 2014, www.cdc.gov/homeandrecreationalsafety/dog-bites/.
2. For more on my training philosophy please visit my website, Good Dog, Happy Baby, www.gooddoghappybaby.com.

Chapter 2. Addressing and Resolving Potential Behavior Problems

1. A helpful overview of the application of antianxiety medications to dog behavior problems can be found online: "Behavioral Medications for Dogs," ASPCA, undated, www.aspca.org/pet-care/virtual-pet-behaviorist/dog-behavior/behavioral-medications-dogs, accessed November 30, 2014.
2. For more information on separation anxiety, please visit my website, Dog Gone Good, www.doggonegood.org.
3. Many "positive only" trainers would take issue with this approach. They would instead suggest doing things like scattering treats across the floor when your dog starts to bark, so that the initial stimulus that got her to

bark becomes associated with treats on the floor — causing her ultimately not to bark but to look for the treats. The result of such an approach is that your dog will learn that barking causes you to throw treats on the floor, and so the behavior will tend to increase rather than decrease. Even if this is not the case, the problem with such an approach is that your dog never learns where the behavior boundary is. In the absence of said treats, she will likely revert quickly to her old behavior.

4. Some dogs are so sensitive that the slightest correction from an electronic collar will send them into a panic. They might respond with a yelp or bark that sets the collar off again, triggering a cycle of panic and pain. This is unusual, but if it happens with your dog, stop using the collar immediately. For such a dog, a citronella collar is the way to go. And if that collar is ineffective, I recommend seeking the help of a professional.

Chapter 3. A Seamless Transition

1. The list is posted on "Snowie's Diary: Dog's Rules of Possession," Dogster, January 5, 2007, www.dogster.com/dogs/227795/diary/Snowies_diary/254395.
2. There are many good trick books available, as well as an almost inexhaustible supply of how-to videos on YouTube.

Appendix

1. There are some interesting online articles about the negative consequences of head collars, including: Suzanne Clothier, "The Problem with Head Halters," Suzanne Clothier Relationship Centered Training, undated, http://suzanneclothier.com/the-articles/problem-head-halters, accessed November 30, 2014; and Roger Hild, "A Not So Gentle Leader," Tsuro Dog Training, undated, www.tsurodogtraining.com/_articles/gentle_leader.html, accessed November 30, 2014.

Index

About the Author

Dog trainer **Michael Wombacher** has performed tens of thousands of private behavioral consultations. An author and lecturer, Mike teaches classes, runs a small boarding and training operation, and trains other trainers. Mike's training approach focuses on channeling a dog's natural drives and instincts into behaviors acceptable in the human pack, primarily by using the principles of positive reinforcement and methods that appeal to the dog's canine sensibilities.

Mike has been certified as an expert on dog behavior by the California Superior Court and does occasional work evaluating dogs in legal matters. He has appeared on numerous television shows, including *Animal Planet*, *Good Day New York*, and *A View from the Bay*, and he has worked with many celebrity clients and prominent tech clients. Mike is a regular contributing writer to *American Dog* magazine, a national publication with a circulation of eight hundred thousand. He currently lives in the San Francisco Bay Area, with his little terrier, Telos. To learn more about Mike, see his websites, DoggoneGood.org and GoodDogHappyBaby.com.

Please visit the Good Dog, Happy Baby online community at

GoodDogHappyBaby.com

You'll find an engaging, evolving community of expecting dog owners and connect directly with author Michael Wombacher. You'll have access to the following features to complement the advice in this book:

A blog

A discussion forum

A video Q&A

Free monthly conference calls

Personalized training consultations

Updated webinars

A comprehensive online video course

For the in-depth Good Dog, Happy Baby video course, visit:

GoodDogHappyBaby.com/good-dog-happy-baby-video-course

This course takes you step by step through some of the most important aspects of preparing your dog for the arrival of your baby. Nearly two years in the making, the course covers content not found anywhere else. With video shot during actual training sessions with dog-owning parents, this course is the next best thing to having Michael in your home training your dog.